Meet Me

∗ ∗ ∗

A Journey Through Pelvic Pain

Amy Watkins

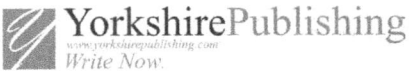

YorkshirePublishing
www.yorkshirepublishing.com
Write Now.

Yorkshire Publishing
3207 South Norwood Avenue
Tulsa, Oklahoma 74135
www.YorkshirePublishing.com
918.394.2665

DEDICATION

If one woman can find comfort in knowing she is not alone, help is available, and strength will find her if she seeks it, then please don't fall into the despair pit, which is a long and ugly way down. If I can offer the hope with belief that help will come for them as well, then I will write this book. I looked but did not find a memoir or self-help book written exclusively by a woman who was plagued herself. The dysfunction is both notoriously unknown and embarrassing. In general, to discuss words like vulva in public is simply not in anyone's best interest. Oh my gosh, I can hardly type the word vulva. It's a horrible word. This body part could have been named something more attractive like "essentia." Medical personnel would then type in patients' charts words like "essentiadynia" or "essentiatherapy" which are quite pleasant to the ear and eye. After all, isn't our pelvic floor essential to life?

Therefore, I dedicate this work of passion to all who want to know more but were either afraid or ashamed to ask, and to those who hold up masks and attempt to pretend all is well. Friends, the issues relative to pelvic floor dysfunction are astonishingly diverse. There may not be enough clinics needed for this area of specialty medicine and therapy. Furthermore, some healthcare providers do not diagnose properly, and do not refer their patients as one might believe they would. For the women who are coping alone, I cannot fathom your suffering. We have created, by our lack of education and shame, an underworld of living survivors of pelvic pain who are unseen in the land of the healthy.

This is dedicated to a healthcare system in reform, to those who stand alongside, and to the thousands of women who are ready for solutions to their pain.

"Such a courageous, honest, and open look at the debilitating physical and emotional effects of chronic pain. The author bears her soul to let others know they are not alone in their feelings - any feelings - especially when it comes to dealing with something as personal as pelvic pain. Kudos to her for breaking the silence and sharing her story of perseverance through this trial."

J. Cole; Author of "Thorns & Roses:
A self-help memoir for women with sexual pain"
Founder of Tulsa Women's Health Alliance

"A vulnerable and personal account that will help women and open the door to communication. While the landscape for persistent pain treatment is improving, diagnosis and treatment options continue to be an uphill battle. Due to its many complexities, treatment takes a team and now this journey will add the writer/patient dimension. Thank you for sharing your story."

Stephanie Prendergast, MPT
Author of "Pelvic Pain Explained"
CEO and Cofounder Pelvic Health and Rehabilitation Center
Los Angeles Branch

"Amy weaves a ribbon of hope through her struggle with pelvic floor dysfunction. Her journey will inspire others dealing with tenacious holds. Yielding control to the pain was not an option for her."

Amy Stein, PT, DPT, BCB-PMD
Author of "Heal Pelvic Pain"
Owner of Beyond Basics Physical Therapy

"A transparent tale of truth. Mesmerizing. Those suffering with chronic pain will find the courage to seek help and a community to support them on their journey."

AJM – anonymous reader

ACKNOWLEDGMENTS

Without the expertise provided by my health team, there would be no story. I am grateful to my physical therapist who diagnosed and treated me for Hypertonic Pelvic Floor Dysfunction. I am also indebted to her physical therapy assistant who guided me to health with patience through her wisdom and knowledge. Thank you both from all of me.

I am also grateful to my acupuncturist who opened a new door of healing. She made it possible for additional relaxation of my extremely tight muscles in body, soul and spirit.

I am thankful for my family and select friends who saw me through by providing empathy, hope, confidentiality and warm embraces. I treasure you. My husband's dedication to the mission of loving me through the pain and allowing me solitude are gifts I cannot repay; free back scratches, for you Mr. Luke, for the rest of my life. I am thankful to God who promises good outcomes to those who wait on the Lord.

TABLE OF CONTENTS

PREFACE

I have no idea what I am doing. Am I writing a diary, journal, or book? When I run out of things to say, will I be cured? If I type faster and write more feverishly, will I gain ground on the final chapter? Am I going crazy at the same time? Whatever it becomes, writing gives me satisfaction. I am doing something constructive, even if only for me. Thoughts which become sentences can then be analyzed, torn apart, shredded, dissected, expanded, or deleted. I am the author of this journey. I can say yes or no to my words. They are mine.

At physical therapy today, Olivia mentioned she had ordered several new books from a holiday gift card. I inquired what books she had purchased; it was a variety of this and that. As things go and because we both enjoyed reading, we discussed a few of the titles more at length. Then Olivia mentioned two books related to treating pelvic floor disorders and my interest was channeled into even more interest but not for the reason she probably thought. The books she had purchased and are now on a shelf six paces away were written by professionals in the field who offer treatment based on medical evidence, new research practices, and patient conferences. The authors had many abbreviated professional degrees to the right of their given names.

Olivia handed one of the books to me and I exclaimed, "I KNEW it!"

She quickly turned her head and asked, "What do you mean?"

I told her emphatically I KNEW the books were written by medical staff but I had yet to find a book written by a woman who had endured and overcome hypertonic pelvic floor dysfunction. Women who research and write their stories on blogs often do not mention their full name out of discreteness. I have found it virtually impossible to find another human being like me.

I then allowed myself to become even more vulnerable; at that moment I was on the therapy table and my muscles were being stretched and encouraged to lengthen. As Olivia also found trigger points, and steadily pressed and held to release their tenacious hold, I disclosed, "I am going to write a book and its title will be: *Meet Me*. Since chronic pain prohibits me from reading more than a few pages at a time, the chapters will be short for those with shortened attention spans due to pain."

And then breathing out, I revealed, "I've already started writing."

My eyes were closed so I couldn't see the expression on her face. I don't know if she was astonished, slightly intrigued, or if she had heard this type of confession before by a previous patient. I don't know if she silently wished me luck or was sad such a book had to be written in the first place. Whatever the cost to myself, I am stepping out for all the other women with me and telling it like it is. This book is for us.

Random Thought:

Am I an accidental tourist in this place of pelvic pain?

In the middle of the journey of our life,
I came to myself within a dark wood,
where the direct way was lost.

- Dante' Alighieri,
Canto 1, Inferno

1
MEET ME WITH A STORY

I t was a cold, wintry night during the holiday season of 2015. Curled up in bed, in a darkened room I read through the night on my tablet. The glow of the screen provided sufficient visibility. I was on winter vacation from my public education career, and had selected another memoir. I am a resource specialist and I love to read. I purchase all genres for students to instill a passion for the written word, but truth be told, I am a realistic genre lover. True events are inspiring with real people who have overcome. My Kindle had recently been replaced by a newer Android tablet. The only reason this is worth mentioning is book covers on a Kindle remain long after a book has been checked back into Overdrive, the e-reader database available through our public library system. This tidbit of knowledge would later haunt me.

That night I read about a female heroine. I don't recall the title or the substance of the book. Sometime after midnight I came to a complete halt. The writer had taken a detour to introduce us to a lady who suffered a malady, the likes I had not ever heard of before. This woman lived in the east and had been bedridden for two years. She had an unimaginable condition and had spoken to few about it. Instead she had resigned her life to lying horizontally and welcomed only a few close friends for visitation. This stricken woman spent her time praying and trying to keep a positive mindset. She could not sit nor walk without intense pain in her groin area. She was not old nor did she have a disease but instead chronic pelvic pain, which was caused by uncooperative muscles. A close friend led her to the revelation of a pelvic pain physical therapy clinic in Arizona. She communicated with the therapist who guided her through the complicated process of traveling hundreds of miles by plane to be seen at the clinic. This was a feat since the woman had hardly left her house in two years. A hotel room was arranged near the clinic and the patient saw the physical therapist daily for a week, and then returned home with an arsenal of tools to manage her life.

I was stunned. My mind was in rapid fire motion with shooting questions. Physical therapy for your vagina? How did she sit in an airplane seat? Why have I not heard of this? How could she be anywhere near positive? Why did she have to go all the way to Arizona? Are there other women who have suffered with this?

I wanted to snap a camera shot of the e-reader page, as it was a monumental discovery for me. This medical predicament was absurd. I could not fathom the inconveniences, pain, and humiliation this woman must have endured. Alas I did not know how to take a screenshot since the tablet was new and I am sort of a slow techie. My cell phone was not on the nightstand. Rousing out of bed to tiptoe into the kitchen to retrieve it was too much of a bother.

"I'll remember," I thought. "I can't possibly forget this. It's too much."

But I did. I have no idea what book I was reading nor why this information was even included in the memoir. All I know is two months later, it happened to me.

2
MEET ME DESPITE A BIOPSY

I had gone in for a regularly scheduled Pap smear on November 18, 2015. I had nothing to fear, just a regulatory thing… only this time it wasn't. Within a week, the OBGYN doctor called me at work; a question had come from the lab. There was something unforeseen that needed to be investigated. It wasn't related to the HPV virus but was possibly a growth that required a biopsy. The prescribed HRT hormone replacement medication needed to be stopped before tests could be done. In fact, I must be off hormones for three weeks.

This telephone call arrived on the day of my early birthday date with Luke, my husband. He had purchased tickets to see a holiday musical out of town. We were excited to attend and did go, but I chose to keep the medical news to myself for a while. This was only a little test anyway.

Unfortunately, my OBGYN, Dr. B was scheduled for surgery the following month and would be turning my case over to a partner, Dr. C or Dr. D. When the nurse called me at work to confirm the details set forth by Dr. C, I flipped out. WHAT DO YOU MEAN OUTPATIENT? Anesthesia? Just great. Now I'll have to share this with Luke, who doesn't need to hear bad news if it's not going to be bad. Emphatically NO. I'm not doing outpatient. Isn't there another option?

"Well," the nurse said, "there was a third physician in the clinic, Dr. D, who performed the same test inside the clinic and anesthesia was not needed." Fantastic! I don't have to miss work for this! "Take some Motrin before arriving," the nurse cautioned.

During my lunch break and before fall semester locker cleanout at school, I arrived at the clinic for the quick biopsy. The doctor had wanted to have a meet and greet beforehand but I had told them that was unnecessary. I wanted to get it over with and I understood the procedure. Upon arrival, I was at ease and the staff was pleasant; I felt comfortable. Positioning myself on the table and into stirrups, I divulged I could endure anything for 15 minutes so he had exactly 15 minutes to get this done. He joked and said, "I am setting my timer and promise to be finished on time."

Four biopsies later and feeling like I had gone into another life dimension of pain and the unknown, I cautiously bent over to put on my pants, and then my sweater top. Outside in the corridor, I walked toward checkout. I presented my paperwork and the receptionist looked at me with wide eyes and awe and said, "You just did all this TODAY?" At that moment, suspended in time, I realized this was not normal. I simply nodded my head in agreement.

I drove myself back to the school. Taking a steel, rolling cart from the supply room, I made my way slowly from one end of the hall to the other, where locker cleanout was about to take place. I am thankful for the brace of the cart which held me up. No one suspected a thing as I became immersed and then camouflaged with the sudden outpouring of 250 students from twelve classrooms who banged and clanged their lockers open and shut. Their task was to find books and objects lost long ago that semester and turn them into me before Christmas break. I rolled the loaded cart back towards my office and then sat in my office chair for the remainder of the afternoon. I don't recall doing another thing but waiting.

3
MEET ME WHEN
THE COAST WAS CLEAR

W aiting.

The phone call that will clear all this misunderstanding about the need for a biopsy. Or four biopsies, in actuality.

"Mrs. Watkins?"

"Yes."

"This is Women's Health OBGYN. Can you hold?"

"Yes."

"Mrs. Watkins? This is Doctor D. You will recall we recently performed a .... (four biopsies in layman's language) and although two came back negative, we are unclear about the other two. We need to have more assurance. When would be a good time to schedule an outpatient, exploratory biopsy?"

Quick. Think. "I believe I have met my deductible for this year (which I hadn't but who cares at this point) so can we do it before December 31st?

"That would work well. Would December 30th be a good date for you, Mrs. Watkins?"

So, with that additional piece of the puzzle my secret was up. I told my husband and daughter, Claire, but asked them to not share it. No need to worry the family during the Christmas celebration, which was to be held in a few days at our house.

There were no complications with the outpatient procedure on December 30th. It did set me back a bit more than I thought it would, however. The next day I wanted to do a little walking at the indoor mall. With Luke's assistance he drove and held my arm as we walked methodically halfway around. I steadily held the pace of an 85-year old woman using a walker. My immediate goals were to put this behind me and move forward.

On January 8th the phone call came from Doctor C (Doctor B and D were unavailable) as expected. The test results showed a "tuft of tissue" in the upper part of my uterus but this was nothing to be worried about. Better safe than sorry, in other words. We would like to see you for a follow-up appointment in two weeks.

At the follow-up, I was told I was healing well; I did feel good. Doctor D stated I could resume sex when comfortable. I reconsidered the HRT medication; since I had now been off it for almost two months was the worst behind me? Would my body continue to adjust and not need hormone replacements? I agreed to wait a few days.

A week later I contacted Dr. C (Dr. B and D were unavailable) and asked to resume hormone medication. Life was too difficult without it.

4
MEET ME THROUGH THE CRITICAL DECISION

I can't do this. I need my estrogen. I telephoned the doctor and asked if he would send in a prescription and he did that same day. However, my body had been without HRT (hormone replacement therapy) for almost two months and I mulled over how soon the symptoms of interrupted sleep, hot flashes, night sweats and crabbiness would begin to subside. In retrospect, it took only two or three weeks for my body to embrace the renewed estrogen level. What I couldn't see was the tissue damage and muscular transformation tipped off from the immediate halt three months prior: the interlude needed for surgery prep and diagnosis. I wouldn't even begin to comprehend the implications of that decision for several more months.

Random Thought:

Have you ever thought that if one thing hadn't happened,
a whole set of things never would've either?
Like dominoes, a single event kicked off an unstoppable
series of changes that gained momentum and spun out of control,
and nothing was ever the same again.
Don't ever doubt that a mere second can change your life forever.

Quotebites.com

5
MEET ME ON ANOTHER SATURDAY NIGHT

Due to family issues and miscommunication we had not yet celebrated my husband's birthday. On February 6th after a nice meal and a few gifts, and it being Saturday and all – aren't couples supposed to have sex on a weekend, especially if it's a birthday weekend? – we had a moment to ourselves. As I opened my eyes the next morning I realized something was extremely wrong. I was on fire "down there." What the HECK? Did I develop a yeast infection in nine hours?

I did what any other woman does in this predicament: I drove to the local pharmacy and purchased the take-this-mess-away ointment, and hoped it would work faster than it said it would on the box. In about three or four days, the burning had subsided and I returned to the gym.

I had started a walking club that launched on January 1st and was determined to not get off track and lose the opportunity to log in miles for the group. We had 33 members and it was an exciting time to be an administrator of a life-changing project. Our name was *The Spatula Sisters* and the motto was "Get out of the Kitchen and Go." My son Liam had created a graphic design, we had business cards, and as the miles from walking, biking, and running began to add up from members month by month, I dreamed this challenge would be inspirational in health benefits as well as provide accountability to not let this challenge slip into a lost New Year's Resolution.

Saturday night rolled around quickly and, being creatures of habit, we snuggled and closed out the day with couple time. Dang it, if the same thing didn't happen again! I awoke Sunday morning with the most intense itching and burning and now I was MAD. What a bad Valentine's Day surprise. My thoughts raced: "What is Luke doing to me? Is he not showering? Is my troublesome hip the problem?"

This time I did not waste time on the ointment but found a vaginal yeast tablet in the medicine cabinet. No change that day or the next. I called my OBGYN and was prescribed more yeast infection tablets to be taken at designated times. I was hopeful.

Nothing changed and this was absurd. Medicine is supposed to work. I made an appointment; upon examination, nothing appeared abnormal. "Have I changed laundry detergent?" I am asked, along with other questions.

"No. No. No."

"Maybe you are dry."

I do have dry skin everywhere else… my legs, my hands, even my eyes don't moisten up well. This is GREAT to find a solution and it's so simple – dry skin! Why didn't I think of that? I am instructed to return to the pharmacy and find a lubricant for feminine dry skin. Have you ever stood in front of the vast array of feminine products and seen the products to help with all kinds of imaginable problems? One must select each product to read the fine print. Is there a time limit for standing in this aisle before you start looking suspicious?

After two weeks of working with this product for "dry skin," all I have is wet panties. I'm still burning and itching like a crazy person. But, of course, I can't itch. Squirming, adjusting, and more bathroom trips are my new normal.

I then cut holes in my panties. I can't stand anything touching my skin.

Another OBGYN consultation. This time we try another ointment with instructions: "Apply several times a day. It has a base that may cause a bit of burning but your insurance will pay for this." OK, I'm up for it. I pay my $25 copay and off I go to the restroom. Immediately my face transforms into a scowl and I begin moaning. "How can this be doing any good when now on top of all the burning and itching, I now have MORE BURNING from this blasted product? What the hell?"

"This is NOT going to work" I tell the doctor the next day. "I'm willing to pay for the cost, even if insurance won't."

I begin to think I am on a lonely road. If a physician believes I can tolerate alcohol-based ointment in an area in which I am dying right now, I am up s*** creek without a paddle.

I'm prescribed a compound instead and wouldn't you know, it is but a brief $5.00 more. My confidence is now running low and my smile is no longer on my face. This month is taking a toll. But I have no other options so I try this new ointment and, success, it does not burn. But what is it supposed to do? The pharmacist tells me it will increase my estrogen level (that was depleted months ago from the "critical decision.")

"Is there a connection between loss of estrogen and this infection with no name?" I wonder.

6
MEET ME INCLUDING
MY NOTEBOOK

March 2011 through June 22, 2016

March 2011: Pap smear by Dr. A – routine

March 27, 2012: Routine checkup by Dr. A. Will change from Microgestin FE 1/20 to Prempro .625/5 next year.

Nov 11, 2013: New prescription for Prempro .625-2.5.

October 31, 2014: Dr. A retires. Routine checkup by Dr. B. "Patient desires to continue original dose of Prempro .625-2.5. HRT benefits and risks reviewed including risks of MI, stroke, breast cancer and VTE."

November 2014: Attempt to refill Prempro .625-2.5 but am told that new prescription of Prempro .3/1.5 is on file. Oh well, I tried. I refill Prempro .3/1.5 instead.

Summer 2015: Two dosages for Prempro are on file at pharmacy. I ask for clarification. Dr. B states Prempro .625 was refilled as requested. Meanwhile, the PA called in the lowest dosage (0.3/1.5) too. We agree to stay on the lower dosage if I am tolerating it well.

November 18, 2015: Routine PAP by Dr. B. No abnormalities. Labia and Vagina normal. My chart says I use Prempro .45-1.5. No documentation of above misunderstanding of the lower dose of Prempro. (I later read pharmacy records and the dose of 0.45-1.5 was not on their file.)

November 24, 2015: Dr. B calls saying my Pap smear came back abnormal with instructions to discontinue using Prempro for upcoming biopsy test.

December 15, 2015: Dr. D performs Colposcopy in the clinic. Endometrial biopsy, endocervical curettage and biopsies were taken. Tests came back inconclusive.

December 29, 2015: Dr. D performs hysteroscopy, D & C with polypectomy and endocervical curettage for AGUS Pap with inconclusive office biopsy showing possible endometrial polyp. The patient's Pap smear showed atypical glandular (abnormal glandular Papanicolaou smear of cervix.)

January 8, 2016: Dr. C post op visit. "Patient states she has severe hot flashes and anxiety. She associates this to the lack of estrogen. She was counseled extensively today about the risks and benefits of hormone replacement therapy. I discussed because of the atypical glandular cells seen on her Pap smear, although endocervical curettage and endocervical curettage were found to be normal, there may still be a lesion present that could be stimulated by estrogen. (Me: MAYBE – all this for MAYBE????)

Findings: Mucus, atrophic endometriu, and a few fragments of benign squamous epithelium and benign endocervical epithelium. Negative for dysplasia, hyperplasic or tumor.

Mid-January: I contact Dr. C and ask to go back on Prempro .3/1.5. I was off hormones for 8 weeks.

February 6: Normal day. Sex with husband that evening.

February 7: Possible yeast infection. Use a vaginal cream and notice a marble-sized inflammation cyst inside my right labia. By February 12th I am almost back to normal.

February 13: Early Valentine sex that evening

February 14: Awaken with horrible itching and burning again. Cold compresses, one Diflucan, and use diaper ointment.

February 19: Dr. B calls in Diflucan 150 mg for one day and then to repeat the dose in 72 hours.

Feb 24: See Dr. B for this "yeast infection" that won't go away. Unclear if symptoms are more vulvar or vaginal. Small amount of drying appearing white d/c. Mild erythema compared to surrounding tissue at fold b/t minora and majora. A vaginal moisturizer is recommended and triamcinolone Acetonide 0.1 ointment is prescribed. Entire lady area severely itches, feels hot, and burns. Wear white cotton panties, no soaps, etc.

March 29: Dr. B office visit. I suspect vulvodynia. Dr. B: "Patients cope a variety of ways, it usually goes away, and is difficult to treat." Exam with Q tip test. When I mention I feel knife cuts in vagina, Dr. B closes the exam immediately. "Is what I said ridiculous or an indicator of something worse?"

I have started the low oxalate diet to see if it will help. Her findings include: no erythema, or lesions at labia, no lesions, no ulcerations, no Lichenifications, 2mm area appears excoriated at clitoral hood where itching was present. Estradiol 0.1 cream is prescribed as a trial – apply to affected area q for 2 weeks, then 1-3x weekly. (A year later, Dr. E prescribed a higher dosage of 0.25grams – 3x per week. I used too low of a dose for 12 months which I believe contributed to atrophy).

March – May: Use Flexeril that was in medicine cabinet. I ask Dr. B and a Dr. F for prescription painkillers for relief and both deny.

Third week of April: I begin to feel better – can sit longer, have more energy, can wear ladies' tap pants style silky undies with dresses. I throw the low Oxalate foods printout away. Good riddance! I celebrate by making a batch of homemade cookies and eat them all.

Last week of April: All symptoms return

Early May: Walk 3 miles on a school excursion. I am apprehensive about what I will wear but my low, slung cotton golf skirt and t-shirt work well. This will be the last long walk I am able to do for over a year.

May 6: Telephone Dr. B and for a referral to the Pelvic Pain Clinic. I now sense tightness, pinching, and aching sensations up inside – more so on my right side. I can no longer lay on my right side. Our conversation closes with "maybe they will teach you some exercises that will help." Not too confident or comforting.

May 15: I lay in bed for a couple of hours that evening, on my back, with this horrible aching in my upper vagina going through my core. If I lay still long enough, I will go to sleep.

May 18: I call my local clinic again. Dr. B prescribes Desipramine 10 mg while I wait to be seen at the Pelvic Pain Clinic.

May 29: Emotional breakdown. I sob in bed, alone, and call out to my husband. "I am so scared, I am so alone, I have so much pain. This thing is taking away who I am until I fear I will no longer be me. I feel like a stick figure that will gradually be reduced to nothing. I would prefer to die than live a life that confines me to bed the rest of my life, living in this pain." Luke asks what medicine he can bring. He is realizing how desperate this situation has become. Later that afternoon, I rouse up and make my way to my secluded hammock, hung between a canopy of trees. I have collected and composed myself, and am comforted by God with this word: "Evie." I message Evie, a friend from the past. I remember she spent time in Eastern culture and learned holistic exercise and relaxation techniques. She battled disease and is strong. "Evie, I'm dealing with a health issue. Can I schedule a time with you? It's complicated and will take a team effort. I believe learning some holistic relaxation techniques is going to help me and whatever other things you have learned."

Evie: Call me anytime (she provides her #)

(I tried to prepare her through text before seeing her in person....)

ME: I am being referred to a pelvic floor specialist but until then am doing my own exercises I have found from a book. On February 7, I developed a horrible problem. The OBGYN first diagnosed it as inflammation but it is much worse than an infection; I begin the search for solutions. Sitting and wearing undergarments are difficult, so I have resorted to wearing big men's boxer shorts and long skirts. Every day I have pain. Cold compress and lying flat are my tools; the doctor has me on some meds, which I am not sure they will work or not. Also laying in my hammock outside is good. This is an unkind condition and although you have great discomfort, you discuss matters within a small community. Only my immediate family and three closest girlfriends know. I hesitate to tell others, as it primarily makes them sad.

Evie: Please allow me to see you tomorrow at your house. Don't put it off. Your situation isn't hopeless. And please do not be ashamed. I do not have to see or touch you naked. We are going to cleanse and relax and reenergize your body. Then your body can help relax, heal, and get well. Let's try. And do not start cleaning your house. I do not care what your house looks like.

THIS WAS THE FIRST TIME I FELT UPLIFTED AND HOPEFUL FOR THE FUTURE IN ALMOST FOUR MONTHS.

May 31 and June 1, 2: Evie came for two hours each morning and we worked on Qigong (an aspect of Chinese medicine), breathing, meditation, removing corruptive thought processes and releasing healing energy within my mind and body. I have not ever experienced a more faithful and loving friend who adjusted her week to minister to me at my deepest need. I will continue many of her practices of meditation, healing my heart, relaxation, cleansing, and use visualization through-out my life.

June 22: First visit to Pelvic Pain Clinic for physical therapy. I lay in the backseat of my husband's F-150 truck with numerous pillows while he drives. I am ecstatic to be seen by professionals who can help. I am also in terrible discomfort. This is the longest 90 miles I have ever driven. I arrive to my appointment in much distress and Dr. Hannah records internal spasms using a timepiece with a second hand, which are con-tracting systematically. She has a phone consult with my new Primary care physician, Dr. G. The OBGYN specialist (Dr. E) is not seeing new patients until August. I will take Baclofen 10 mg and Tizanidine 4 mg. to calm spasms.

And that's my story or, in reality, the beginning of it. Please con-sider this your invitation to Meet Me on my Journey Through Pelvic Floor Dysfunction.

7
MEET ME AND I MEAN ALL OF ME

' **P**elvic pain' is a moderately vague term that is confusing to many. Questions arise such as are you talking about the hips or the pelvis bones? Are you referring to the belly area below the navel? Are you describing pain as in childbirth? Some women might be thinking, does this refer to sensations from infections such as bacterial vaginosis or a yeast infection? Or is this term used more broadly to highlight bladder issues such as urinary tract infections and even possible kidney stones? A more generalized question might be, "Are we communicating about the inside or the outside of the body?" Is this a sexual issue or more of a digestive tract malfunction?

"Friends, all the above."

This is a complicated muscular, skeletal, and nerve ending relationship with no known cause but several theories have surfaced: hormonal fluctuations, injuries – subtle and severe – infections, and many other inconclusive ideas.

In retrospect, I have held a lot in and used up my reserves. I must say goodbye, fare thee well to anything that causes lower abdomen clenching. This would include saying yes to many restroom breaks instead of "holding it," no shivering will be allowed, and I'll forevermore wear layered clothing. I will be cautious about traveling. I want to travel, don't get me wrong. But I may have to limit the number of hours I can physically sit in a vehicle. I will be disappointed if I cannot ever ride my bike again. Did you know a variety of bicycle seats to accommodate both men and women now have crevices like the Grand

Canyon cut down the center to prevent damage to sensitive areas? I purchased one of these classy, ostentatious new seats and do have high hopes. But if I can't ride, I will accept it.

Without naming body parts, think of the front of the groin area as north I35 as it runs to the hip area, which is south I35 in the DFW area (Dallas/Fort Worth). Pelvic pain ran the line of I35 but was most severe on the I35E interstate that divided away from the Dallas course. Others will attest to different experiences but they are all private, unspeakable, and even my daughter Claire, who is a registered nurse, advised, "Mom, this is not dinner conversation." But it is necessary to speak freely with your health providers about the specifics or you will not make headway. It does help to have a female clinician but when you have Chronic Pelvic Floor Dysfunction, the lines of male and female providers merge. You want expertise, period.

I have been told by my team that help is long in coming for some patients because they are embarrassed to seek help or do not know where to turn. Some patients have suffered many years before they made their first medical appointment. I cannot fathom this. Maybe their pain was not as severe as mine. At my latest massage, the therapist told me she had worked on a client who had similar issues as mine. The client normally went to another massage therapist in the spa but because she was unavailable, the client was seen by the one I use.

The therapist asked her, "Have you seen a medical doctor for this?"

"No, I have no idea who to go to," replied the woman.

I have discovered for myself when you have this kind of private issue that affects so many muscles, which makes simple living almost inconceivable some days, you do not trade around with therapists unless it is unavoidable. They learn to know your body, your muscles, which ones are extra tight and so forth. You do not want to keep repeating your same medical history over and over to new people, which is exhausting and humiliating. When my therapist saw this new client, and read her history to learn of her area of concern and the techniques utilized to alleviate pain, she immediately thought of me.

I asked my therapist, "How long has this woman been coming for treatment?"

She replied, "Two years."

That was discouraging to me. From a legalistic viewpoint with medical practices and violations, her name would not be divulged so that I might offer my insight. Maybe this woman gets relief with weekly massages and can function in her daily life and does not need additional physical therapy techniques, but I doubt it. Two years is a long time. How many thousands of women are trying to get by the best they know how?

My daughter Christine called me excitedly one day, "Mama I just passed a billboard which was advertising Carrington Memorial Hospital. It said: Come to Us for Pelvic Floor Disorders." Word is getting around in the big city but in my area of the world, still taboo.

Well, I'm speaking out. "Meet me and I will go through this with you."

Random Thought:

I am ready to proceed in a new direction.

8
MEET ME READING BLOGS

I began to scour the Internet to discover what the heck was going on. Researching was my lifeline to answers I knew would be flowing in from others. Women spoke openly with what they were dealing with, their coping skills, recommendations for healthcare providers, medications that worked and those that did not, and their own private experiences. I spent hundreds of hours researching, reading blogs, and learning new terminology as I retrained my brain to understand female anatomy. I was astounded by how little I knew. I had NEVER heard of so many complications related to basic body functions that affected both women, men, and children.

Incredibly, oxalate is a relatively new medical finding that can account for intense kidney and urinary malfunctions and is found in food that comes from the garden and trees! It can create serious burning effects while urinating. Oxalate crystals can be excreted through pores and ducts, causing rashes and painful eye blinking. Bowel movements have a different consistency with oxalate and the vagina can also be affected with burning pain. Upon general inspection, not even an examining physician can see a darn thing. It's like a phantom disease.

Another frightening anatomical phenomenon is the entrapment of the pudendal nerve. This nerve wraps from the base of the spine and divides like a milkweed root system which, in the case of a healthy system, regulates bowel movements and works with nerve and motor support systems. However, one becomes alarmed with the potential pain and suffering associated with this invisible area near the tailbone when the pudendal nerve is entrapped. More words like neuralgia, neuropathy, nerve blocks and the dreaded surgery will jump directly from the computer screen and embed themselves in the memory crevices of your brain. Renowned specialists practice in a minority of locations around the world. If you believe you have a problem with your pudendal nerve, this is a problem, with a capital P.

How about our sisters in battle who we meet online who live in the UK, Canada, and other continents of the world? They are suffering! And they are oftentimes suffering alone. One young lady reached out to say she had been bedridden for over two weeks. When she tried to get up, she was in agony that resonated throughout her entire core. I have so many questions about these ailments. Ask twenty ladies what they believe the functions of the pelvic floor are, and they will provide twenty different answers – discreetly, of course.

I was advised to stay away from researching excessively. "You don't need the negativity," they said, and, "you might be given wrong advice." I nodded in agreement that I didn't need any more negativity but didn't buy into this philosophy. I instead began to take notes, ask questions, and gained knowledge to speak more clearly with physicians about therapies and medications. Without my research, I doubt I would have been placed on two medications that were not initially prescribed. I had not been advised to use acupuncture but instead found my own clinic. It was a continual quest to find various seat cushions that provided a bit of relief. I read articles from medical journals and purchased books online dealing with chronic pelvic pain. "In fact, would I have been referred to the Pelvic Pain Clinic at all if I had not asked Doctor B.?"

Studies show if you write 750 words per day it increases creativity, articulation, and purpose. Writing allows your thoughts to flow and ultimately have a record of them. In fact, check it out: 750words.com. I will write. I will learn about myself. I will express my deepest and most twisted and painful thoughts in the hopes I will get redemption and validation that this dysfunction was REAL. I had a life of many compromises due to pain and inability that the scope was beyond description. Writing will erase any future doubt that this season of life was too harsh of a memory and that I acted irrationally. I pledge not to forget but to move forward.

Random Thought:

My new friend is a heating pad but my best resource is finding peace.

9
MEET ME ON THE NAMING COMMITTEE

I'm not sick. I'm not healthy. I don't have a disease. I don't have a terminal illness. I don't have a measurable fever. My bloodwork is excellent. My blood pressure is admirable. My heart is pumping, I'm alive, but I feel bad.

I'm also a little mad. Why didn't they give this condition a real name with substance? I simply have a dysfunction. Who is on the naming committee for medical conditions? I believe it must have been a man who named this 'Pelvic Floor Dysfunction'. A woman would have insisted on a name that described the agony in rich detail. A dysfunction is the best you can do? We all have dysfunctions. My blower dryer for my hair doesn't always come on. I occasionally have diarrhea. My nose drips when I eat spicy food. Those are dysfunctions.

No, this is not a dysfunction. If I had been on the naming committee, here are my ideas.

Labor Contractions That Last for Months Syndrome

Muscles Being Pulled out by Aliens from the Vagina Misery

Weird Pellets Under Your Skin That Cramp but Weren't There Before Plague

Sitting in Hot Oil and Can't Get out of It Mania

The Invisible Nightmare that Won't Go Away Abnormality

The No Marathon but Feels Like It Anyway Affliction

The No Surgery Malady

The Attack out of Nowhere Infirmity

My Legs Feel Like a Squeezed Tube of Toothpaste Secret

Women Hiding in Pain Malfunction

In my opinion, the Naming Committee messed up big time on this one. They didn't have the courage to call it for what it is.

Random Thought:

This oxalate diet is terrorizing me! Items on the "good" list are all meats. Just great; I'm a balanced eater which to me means high on fruits and veggies, part Mediterranean, part Mexican and Italian, and peanut butter sandwiches.

If I was to succeed at eliminating oxalates from my pores, tissues, and all crevices from my body, I must understand and follow this diet with consistency. Out went the wheat, potatoes, and white rice, and two thirds of the veggies and fruit. Modest amounts of a few variety of nuts were okay as were a limited list of fruit tea. It was exhausting to shop. During one grocery trip I purchased over $100 worth of items for Luke but was so rattled with confusion that I came home with only one item for me! I became scared to eat.

Even after Dr. Q emphasized with authority that my dysfunction involves muscles that pull, which leads to intense burning and discomfort, I was afraid she might be wrong. I was trapped in this diet for five months and it took many more months before I could enjoy another peanut butter sandwich again.

10
MEET ME IN BED

Married people sleep together, or are supposed to, in the same bed. Several years ago, due to sinus issues and snoring, teenagers who kept late hours, and my light sleeping status, this was no longer possible. I tried different things such as using ear plugs and moving to the couch when I was awakened during the night. But my back hurt from sleeping on the sofa. I started to resent the whole situation and eventually gravitated to sleeping in the now spare bedroom after the last teenager moved away from home. Yes, this caused some issues and we both felt a rift developing at times, but when you are going on less than optimal sleep any misunderstanding can get out of hand in a split second. We both adjusted and as time went on, came to accept the situation. In case you are wondering, we still had couple time… that is, up until February 2016. With an uncertain diagnosis, pelvic pain, and fear on both our parts of exasperating the situation, we both agreed to wait.

When this condition happened without warning, we were already adjusted to sleeping alone. Thank Heavens! Oh my goodness, I had to develop new solutions and quick. Being married for 30 plus years lends itself to healthy communication but I wasn't ready to open the doors to share all the details of this predicament I had suddenly found myself in. For instance, during the early part of this journey I kept a tall glass of iced water on the bookshelf next to the bed. On fiery evenings, that cold glass would rest in between my legs to cool the area off so I could then go to sleep. I kind of froze myself into a non-feeling zone. About the second month with vulvodynia, Dr. B asked if I had freezer burned myself, so that had turned out to be a bad idea. The ointments and creams, and pillows, the heating pad, the weighted pillows, the fleecy blanket, the TENS machine, all the cords – well, you can see sleeping alone was best for both of us. Not to mention using the Therawand. Tentatively and in secret under the sheets, this strange device, which was coated with dripping lubricant, was used to stretch out the insides since we were no longer having sex. Something needed to keep the doors opened down below and there was no way sex was going to be happening.

Sleep.

This was the one time my body was at peace with itself. I slept with the door closed and a nightie eye shield to block out any light. Sleep was my haven and I relished it.

Random Thought:

Is this going to be a forever thing?

11
MEET ME AT THE LIQUOR STORE

Growing up, my family did not stock liquor in our home, nor did my parents ever drink it. My mom recalled sipping champagne in the streets as neighbors celebrated after WWII was declared over. I had tried drinking a taste of this and that as a teenager but had not experienced the true pleasure others did, or so they pretended. It tasted awful. I was more of the Dr. Pepper with a shot of vanilla and cherry, with a squirt of chocolate syrup kind of girl.

The 20's, the 30's, the 40's, the 50's and whoa... My mindset changed.

I was in agony and didn't know where to turn. The only thing our medicine cabinet held of any value to me were muscle relaxers my husband had needed when extending his right shoulder in a golfing tournament. It was either those or Nyquil. I took the muscle relaxers until they ran out. I then called Dr. B and the nurse reported they wouldn't be prescribing any pain or anxiety medications and to see my primary care physician instead. My PCP was one of my husband's best friends and there was NO WAY I was making an appointment to visit about this new development between my legs. I opted for a phone call to his nurse instead. I began to tell her my issues and then started to sob. In a gentle manner, she assured me that she would speak to Dr. F right away. "Could I come in this afternoon?"

"No, I don't need to come in; there is nothing to see."

A prescription would be called in right away then. That was comforting to have an alliance. But what was called in were more muscle relaxers; no anxiety and no pain medication. "Disappointed" is not the word I felt but at best a bit relieved to have a vial of muscle relaxants to send me into sleep – a welcome distraction from my living hell.

With great resolve, a pair of sunglasses, an ID, and a quick trip to the liquor store I purchased several six packs of assorted wines. I prayed to the highest heavens I wouldn't run into anyone I knew! I didn't care if I saw them but I sure didn't want them seeing ME in a liquor store. Any explanation would sound perfunctory. I was in and out in 5 minutes, had the goods, and felt like I had pulled off a heist. This makes no sense to 90% of Americans but to me it was a big deal to begin consuming wine at this stage in life. I was out of options so I geared up into survival mode then waited for relief and a referral to a specialist. No lasting relief came, but eventually a referral did.

For some odd reason, I felt it was important to keep those little bottles. I washed them out and stored them in sacks at the back of my closet. I love glass artwork and one day it occurred to me that these little bottles would become part of my healing process. I could paint each one, adorn them in tiles or dazzling jewels, and then showcase them together as a trophy piece, a bottle tree that would provide beauty in the wake of this terrible year of uncertainty and pain. Yes, I could do that.

12
MEET ME UNDER THE UMBRELLA

A t the top of my body is my head. On my head are visible protru-
sions and accessories, if you will, that to you may or may not
seem attractive, noteworthy, or even worth mentioning. On heads, one
generally sees hair or the lack of it, two eyes, two ears, one nose, one
mouth, and a chin. Upon further examination, other facets are revealed
such as the color of your tongue, scars, or possible areas that may need
to be seen by a specialist. The skeletal feature holds the head together
and we can assume that a working brain, which coordinates the tiniest
balances of the, is functioning well. We don't see them, but we know
muscles are holding the eyes in their sockets, connective tissue runs
through our sinus passages, and nerve endings scream OUCH when we
get a bad sunburn after a day at the beach.

The head is full of it. So much goes on in the head. Skeletal, muscular, neurological, emotional sensations, and blood. Plenty of it (blood)
is circulated back and forth, providing a working and sensational piece
of art we call the human body. Slight discomforts such as a sore throat,
a nosebleed, ear infection or a migraine headache are involved in this
thing called "the head." The more serious aspects of medical technologies involving the removal of tumors, the managing of seizures, and the
subconscious aspects of taking a breath, one after another without even
thinking about it are done in the head. The head is a big thing.

This is the way I have come to terms with my Pelvic Floor
Dysfunction. In my pelvic area are bones, connective tissues, nerve
endings, and multiple muscular fibers that overlay, hold up structures,
and provide highways from one organ to another so the core of my

body is held in shape and can move freely. Blood flow, communication with one another, and range of motion are key elements to this area's effectiveness.

When Googling Pelvic Floor Dysfunction, a litany of disorders and discomforts will pop up for your inspection. Experts agree Pelvic Floor Dysfunction is an umbrella for many pathologies that oftentimes co-exist together within one individual. The list is exhaustive: intestinal obstruction, diverticulitis, urinary tract infection, irritable bowel syndrome, pain associated with ovulation, pelvic inflammatory disease, symphysis pubis dysfunction, ovarian cysts, appendicitis, ovarian torsion (twisting of the ovary), ectopic pregnancy, pelvic congestion syndrome, endometriosis, vulvodynia, bacterial vaginosis, and pelvic floor tension myalgia. Let's not forget interstitial cystitis, vestibulodynia, coccydynia, anismus, prolapse, uterine fibroid tumors, bowel and bladder issues, and sexual dysfunction.

Data collected agrees that 15-32% of women will have a Pelvic Floor Dysfunction. www.nichd.nih.gov "How many women have pelvic pain?" by Eunice Kennedy Shriver, National Institute of Child health and Human Development. Another study found that 12-20% of women experience chronic pelvic pain and about 61% of the cases go undiagnosed. * U.S. News and World Report. "Origin of chronic pelvic pain in women can be elusive." January W. Payne, March 8, 2010.

It's like comparing three women who played softball. One slid into home base and ripped the skin off her elbow to her wrist. It will heal, but it hurts so much it dominates all senses and she needs immediate wound care. The second woman collided with another player and broke her arm. She is having trouble moving at all; everything hurts. X-rays are ordered, surgery is scheduled, and the arm will be in a cast for two months. The third person on the team dislocated her shoulder and considering that this is a reoccurring injury, she is out of the game. No more softball for her. But wait, someone in the stands has come to cheer on a loved one. It was a gorgeous day and why not experience life by being involved and relishing all it offers? There she sat in the bleachers when up went a fly ball, propelling itself downward at 110 mph and with no warning struck the head of the spectator, who had turned her eyes from the game for a few moments to catch a conversation with a friend. The ball struck her in the right spot which resulted in residual damage. She will need therapy, encouragement and motivation, and will also require new coping skills to conquer daily tasks that yesterday she did with ease. Poor lady, all she wanted to do was attend a ball game!

It was a head injury, and it falls under the same umbrella as "something is not right in my head." Levels of discomfort in the head range from tonsillitis to permanent disability in this long list of things you would prefer not to happen. The list is too long and the umbrella is too wide.

This categorization makes as much sense to me as being told that up to 32% of women will have Pelvic Floor Dysfunction. The list is too long, the therapies too varied, the solutions which may help for some, but not for all, are not substantiated for total agreement by even the specialists. The growing number of professionals who manage the range of pain levels caused by this dysfunction is mind blowing. What a highly individualized matter for EACH patient this is which lends itself to such disparity. I am now in this percentage group with the assignment of hypertonic pelvic floor muscles and I don't know one person with these peculiarities, and I know a lot of people.

13
MEET ME AMONG THE BON TEMPS

C ecelia, Lila, and Sarah are three special friends of mine, and we are members of the Bon Temp Sisterhood. Our earliest history unfolds at Baylor, specifically inside Collins Dormitory. When we each moved in, three of the four knew no one. To get acquainted and make friends that first month there were many activities on campus, as well as planned events in each dorm. One evening, it was announced there would be an upcoming meeting in the main drawing room for all residents. The purpose was to form new friendships and to also find travel partners so freshmen without transportation could travel home occasionally on weekends. I had a car and was more than willing to fill it with others to help share the cost of mileage. What was I thinking? It was only 57 cents a gallon but then the cost of living was reduced as well. I guess it all evened out.

At the Meet Your Neighbors meeting I met two lovely girls from my own hometown. Ironically, both had attended the same HUGE high school but had not met, not ever having classes together or probably the same lunch period either. They were from the northside and I was from the southside. You wouldn't think our experiences would have varied much, living 20 miles away, but in hindsight I can see we were as different as night and day. Nevertheless, we clicked. Down the same hall from me lived a third new friend whom I would also grow to love.

Baylor was a magical place. As we reminisced years later, "Youth is wasted on the young" – George Bernard Shaw. We had no idea how blessed we were to receive an education that was affordable, live among beautifully designed buildings with so much history and culture, and the food – delicious and homemade with ice crystal sculptures brought in and used as centerpieces during extravagant Friday night buffet nights. We developed strong ties all over the United States as well as from Europe and South America. Our world was opening and stretching.

Through the years, the four of stayed in touch, rooming with one another some, carpooling, sharing, eating, living, laughing and sometimes crying with one another. The years ran together and during our 2005 get-together, we christened ourselves with a name. We were in New Orleans at the time: a city filled with culture, music and fun. The motto for New Orleans is "Laissez les bon temps roulez" – a Cajun expression meaning "let the good times roll!" It conveys the "joy of living," an attitude that pervades south Louisiana (Urban Dictionary). Four cheers and a toast later, we were four girls with a new name. We were the Bon Temps.

The Bon Temps have kept me going in more ways than one this year. I hesitated to let them know too much, as their lives were a mixture of fun, travel with husbands, entertaining guests, serious business, finances, responsibilities connected with grown children, parents, siblings, you name it – we all had issues. I didn't want to add more woe. I wanted to continue to add "wow" but this was not to be my wow year. I kept them afloat with basic things I was experiencing but, finally, I let down my hair and let them see the real me - the struggling me who was barely making it some days.

Not losing sight of our goal of friendship through thick and thin, they rallied by sending cards, typed many emails, sent prayers on my behalf, and mailed care packages with thoughtful gifts I cherished. I tried to remain hopeful, but honestly there were days that were just too much. I would write an email to them and then often delete it before pressing "send." They were my sisters but I didn't want to cause unnecessary worry. I had learned my bad days weren't EVERY SINGLE stinking day and once a thought is written and sent, it stays in the mind of the receiver. So I pretended a lot and, to be honest, that was beneficial to all of us. Who can be around a complaining, afraid, hopeless sounding individual for long? I didn't even want to be around myself some days!

Instead, I soaked up their optimism and good-feeling-vibes that I read from each through daily emails and lived somewhat vicariously through them. Seeing life from a different perspective is enlightening. Traveling to new spots, experimenting with new recipes and trying new restaurants, hosting events and visiting with neighbors and friends kept the world in balance for me. Most of the time I was home alone but I didn't feel isolated. I could envision them with their conversational husbands, attending a painting class, tutoring a student, caring for an elderly relative, or restoring a part of their home, and I was included. It felt good to have my eyes opened and I was conscious of the tinkling of a dream that I, too would one day join their circle of activity as my body renewed itself over the next year.

Random Thought

My world is shrinking but I don't know that I have missed anything truly important.

14
MEET ME AS I HANG ON

I trust You. I believe in You. There must be a plan, a reason. This isn't random. I am not a mistake. You will make it so.

Trust. Only five letters but a BIG word. Especially when you don't have much.

T R U S T

T R U S

T R U

T R

T

Somedays, I can only hang on to the letter T. One simple letter. But I am still hanging on.

When given the following statement: "I just found out I have xxxxx and will be undergoing intensive treatment for six months. Hopefully that will take care of it." What do you say?

a. "I'm so sorry to hear this""""

b. "What can I do for you?"

c. "I would like to check in on you weekly if you don't mind."

d. Answers A, B, and C

e. "Thank God it's only 6 months!"

NEVER say: "It's only 6 months." You have no idea how long six months can be.

15

MEET ME AT THE PELVIC PAIN CLINIC

I was overcome when the receptionist told me I was scheduled for June 22nd for my first physical therapy appointment. My voice broke and tears flowed when I shared the good news with Luke. I was elated. I marked PT in big letters on the kitchen calendar. There had been good intentions for getting me in sooner but a referral delay from my local OBGYN clinic had cost me two or three additional weeks. I waited impatiently for confirmation. I faxed my profile myself. I could not believe healthcare was so slow. I was extremely uncomfortable every waking second; this put me in a sour frame of mind. My activities were diminishing; chronic pain insists you view your new world through a narrow straw. I had a severe case of tunnel vision.

Now that I was scheduled, I read up on what to expect and attempted to complete the packet of information that was mailed to me. I procrastinated. The packet was thick and the more I looked at the manila envelope, the more fearful I became. I was to bring it with me, completed, to my first appointment. I waited until a few days beforehand to see what they wanted to know.

Oh my, the questions. I was now in unfamiliar territory. The documents were professional, concise and held detailed information that both reassured and terrified me. I worked on the medical profile for several hours. I had not thought in these terms with questions such as: "What is your pain level while carrying a bag of groceries from the car into your home? Do you refrain from attending events with friends?

How far can you walk: a few yards, one block, half a mile?" On and on it went.

June 22nd arrived and I was to be here 15 minutes prior to my appointment. Luke and I arrived 45 minutes ahead of schedule. Traveling 90 miles with traffic, we might encounter a number of delays: car wrecks and rerouted highway closures were part of city life. There was no way I was going to miss this appointment due to traffic.

The clinic was modern, beautiful, and larger than I expected with seven floors comprised of various types of specialized medical care. With determination, I boarded the elevator, pressed the 7th floor button, and entered the Pelvic Pain Clinic. I turned over the paperwork and was invited to take a seat. I politely smiled and replied, "Thank you." Luke had driven while I lay in the backseat atop firm sofa cushions from our sectional at home. Every bounce and jiggle of the car sent penetrating spasms into my core area and sitting compounded the problem. So, instead, I walked to the foyer with beautiful foliage and floor to ceiling glass windows overlooking the city. I held onto the banister. My pulse was out of control and I was on the verge of a panic attack. Breathe in, hold, and breathe out. Over and over. Eyes closed. Center yourself. Hold on.

I had envisioned a crowded waiting room filled with sad women, standing for the sake of sitting. No one would be wearing slacks. Sullen husbands would sit isolated from another in their own private thoughts. I would be thrust into stirrups while indifferent doctors, therapists, and general onlookers in training would come in and out, examine every inch of my body, make comments, and whisper as they logged obscene things they saw about my body. I knew the door would swing open often and I would feel violated. I envisioned being naked, cold, and shivering without a sheet for an hour as they would leave me stranded in a patient room due to appointments running far behind schedule. I knew I had to come but it was no doubt going to be the most undesirable, humiliating, and painful experience I would ever have.

I couldn't have been more wrong about my expectations.

My name was called and I entered and, again to my surprise, was greeted with a concerned and loving woman. I will always remember her kindness and intentional conversation with eyes directed at me as I told her my story. Dr. Hannah had read my paperwork and the fax of the "story of my recent life" I had provided in desperation. I needed help and they would be my route out of this horrible nightmare that had begun on February 7th. She empathized, sympathized, verified, and gave me hope. After her evaluation and recommendations for a medical plan, she considered my question, "How long will I have this pelvic problem?"

Dr. Hannah replied, "I believe you will see results in six to twelve months." My eyes teared up and my face fell. Understandably she reached out to touch my arm and with tenderness said, "I believe it is possible you will return to normal within a year but it all depends on many factors."

I stifled my sobs and regained my composure. "I am not crying because it is going to take so long. I'm crying because this isn't going to be permanent."

After an hour and a half of professional care, I left with hope. Two prescriptions would be called in and a plan for lengthening tight muscle constrictions was in place. Dr. Hannah claimed she and Olivia, the physical therapy assistant, love their patients, and I was refreshed. Later I would reflect upon that statement. This would be the first time a physician would vocalize to me that their medical team loves their patients. In hindsight, I now understand because pelvic floor therapists are directly involved in recovery and see patients a considerable amount of time, the medical community sometimes knows little about the specialized care they provide. The number of hours the three of us would eventually spend together would constitute a true and lasting relationship between friends.

Random Thought:

I find myself looking with longing at the clinic's yoga ball. I will relish every bit of progress I make!

16
MEET ME AND THE
IMPRESSION OF WORDS

Words are powerful, liberating, creative, encouraging, informative, and provide an escape. Words also have the power to harm and to be discouraging when coming from a negative mind and heart. I'm finding that the written word sustains me. Positive. Words. Speak. In craft stores and home décor boutiques, decorative and powerful words are all over. People need visualization of the power of words. We all need to be reminded we are not alone and have a community. Printed on canvas, engraved in stone, and molded into all types of materials from rod iron pieces to ceramic, cloth, and paper.

Words: written on scraps of paper, held together in book bindings, printed on magazine and newspaper headlines, and countless other written communication possessions we all come across. We don't often take advantage of their full potential. With a desire to slow down my pace of life and to find a higher meaning through the highs and lows, the written word stands out as an epic form of sensory detail that is both helpful but desirably one of the single most points of making or breaking a thought pattern. Words will help me to live on a higher plane.

Words. In the English language, 26 letters are used to create manuscripts worth millions, which are displayed in museums. Twenty-six letters also create passages of love and warmth written in beautiful language for lovers and snuggled together mamas and babies. Pinterest, Etsy, and other social media icons have brought the written word to a whole new access level with easy maneuvering within the Internet to find the right quote to convey our soul's deepest desires even when we are inadequate to express journal type entries ourselves.

I also grasp hold of the written word through scripture. Reading passages from the Bible on subjects of fear, joy, and protection have been beneficial. I meditate and words come to me that help to calm my mind and anatomical nervous system. I'm plain out of balance, and without seeking words of healing, I would have no hope.

On a new medication handout prescribed to help deal with pain were the following words: "This medication was prepared specifically for you." In the past, I wouldn't have even read the accompanying literature. This line resonated with me and I reread it often throughout the week. "Specifically, for me." That phrase gave me peace of mind that my medical team was there for me. Me. I'm not a number, but a real person who needs their attention and direction. This new life path is too confusing. I need help from others. "Thank you," I whisper back.

Random Thought:

Beauty and Joy are all around. I have forgotten to look. I must search more intently.

17
MEET ME AS I JOIN A GROUP

The moderator of this online group invited the newest members to introduce themselves. We were assured we would find a community of support.

"Hello, I'm Amy. I'm all for positive thoughts and friendship along this road to healing!" I then shared my background starting with the abnormal Pap, discontinuing estrogen, outpatient surgery, possible infection, confusion, pain, and the realization I now had vulvodynia. I included what I had tried, including medications, clothing changes, stress reduction, various seat cushions, and mentioned I had recently started pelvic floor therapy. In retrospect, I divulged a bit too much on this "first date" with thousands of people, but I was frantic to find anyone who had experienced my symptoms and then gained relief. I was hoping to find a cure, if truth be known. I ended by writing I had the endurance and discipline to see this through and believed God had a plan for me through this. I then invited others who would like to be encouraging path walkers in this journey to contact me via email.

Within days, I opened my email account and there it was; one person had responded to my inquiry. My first pen-pal/pelvic pain sister. She and I were surprised only one had replied but were thankful to have found each other. Thus, we began a six month, moving friendship that inspired me to keep going.

I will be forever grateful for her kind heart, her open soul, and her desire for a spiritual sister to share the journey with her just as I was needing. We openly spoke about all aspects of our lives and became fast friends. We emailed consistently and although I was still working and received about 50 emails daily, hers was the first one I read. She was my mentor, confidant and spiritual advisor. I soaked up her words and encouraged her to write her story as she had such a strong message and style. We went through the seasons of summer, fall and winter together. We laughed and celebrated humble victories. We encouraged one another. She indeed was my lifeline and not only held my hand through the miles but also held my heart in place as it protested, grieved and feared. Thank you for walking the journey with me, sweet sister.

Random Thought:

Offering empathy is so important. I once thought it was sympathy which was needed but the two are vastly different. Empathy is the glue that connects one to another.

18

MEET ME AFTER THE BABY POWDER DANCE PARTY

"Go see what the children have done," Claire said with a mischievous smirk.

"Where are they?" I asked.

"Oh, you will know! Just go down the hallway."

A few steps later, my nose picked up a familiar fragrance. As I peered into the youngest one's bedroom, I stopped dead in my tracks. What had been a vibrant splash of bright pinks with celery and forest green accents was now masked in white. Powder hung suspended in the air. All furniture surfaces had a dusting of white. The carpet had taken the biggest hit and was saturated in white stuff. Little fingers had run through it – had the little ones tried to make snowballs? The sphere of influence had also spread into the opened closet doors. All the dresses, sweaters, and two-piece outfits dangling on the clothes rack would need to be laundered again. The air was pungent. Although the little ones had been reprimanded by their mommy, they were still proud of their work. "Look what we did, Ama!" they squealed in delight.

Claire had enlisted their help in the clean-up process but right away realized that it was a bad choice. The layers of powdery white were getting smeared out even more. Plus, the hazy air had set off allergy symptoms. Oh, where to start?

This assailant disguised as a bottle of baby powder is an object lesson for chronic pelvic pain. How could a household product, for babies no less, become so ill-fated? Or with creative license, can we ask, "How then can pelvic muscles created for structural foundation and digest and elimination that feed the entire body then sabotage this area so fiercely?" Chronic pain is a trial and tribulation, a burden that creates stress and is an un-fun problem to have. Chronic pain encases multiple challenges. Just as a baby powder dance party, the areas affected are so numerous, one might not know where to start in making things right again. Until you've been there, you won't believe its workload and the stretch of time required for this liability. This affliction is a burdensome task that calls us to duty with diligence to rid ourselves of this pain in the ass.

Powder had gotten into the children's hair, was caked on their arms, and stuck to areas between toes where the skin was damp. It was either lightly resting or piled high on every horizontal surface in the room. The smell burned our sensitive eyes. This was no average mop up, spruce up, tidy up, or even wipe up type of task and would prove to live up to the definition of a chore! It couldn't be ignored nor would it go away on its own. This was not a task for the faint of heart nor those wanting an easy way out. Commitment with a purpose-driven focus was the solution to get this room back to a livable condition, which was the first goal in sight. And commitment with a purpose-driven focus was the only way to get MY body back to a livable condition, which was my first goal, also.

Random Thought:

If an obstacle is on the road ahead, I don't steer straight into it but look beyond the threat; safe driving demands that I maneuver around while still moving forward.

19
MEET ME IN COMMANDO MODE

Wearing panties was the norm. I put them on after a shower and they stayed on. I took them off to change, but another pair went right back on. I slept with panties. To not would have been unnatural. Too open. I did go skinny dipping once (with Luke) just to say we did it. That felt both odd and free in the middle of the lake with only a life preserver. But that had been in fun.

Going without panties is now necessary and I mean COMPLETELY necessary. No fabric can touch. I wear long skirts and slips and pray to the highest heavens that I'm not in a car wreck, not for fear of injury to myself or my car, but I am apprehensive about something else. Being sent to the hospital by ambulance, the staff might cut off my skirt or dress and then call out to one another in surprise, "Hey, this lady isn't wearing panties!"

It didn't start off that way. I graduated backwards. First, I cut out a slit in the cotton panty to give more breathing room. Then I made the slit larger, much larger, until it was in fact a huge hole. "OMG, is this even called a panty anymore?" I refused to let my husband touch my laundry. How do you even start to process holding up a pair of panties with half of them cut out?

Then I moved onto XL men's white cotton boxer shorts. I had read that fabric dye may cause irritation. So huge, unladylike white boxer shorts it was. I wore these essential elements under conservative length dresses and skirts. If I had leaned over or a gust of wind had blown a shortened hemline up, my boxer shorts would have been exposed. I can't even think about it! Sadly, even boxer shorts became uncomfortable. The perception of a "wedgie" intensified with the light touch of fabric. I could not afford to exasperate this problem which ran from the right side of my navel, down through the groin and then up again throughout my right butt cheek. The awareness of a drawstring cinched up in this invisible line was maddening.

As my options shrunk, my resolve grew. I bought a thong; certainly such a tiny thing would not cause too much havoc. Wrong! That thong was ripped off in 30 seconds flat. Then came ladies' boy shorts, bigger than my normal size but soft in texture and feminine in a way. I got two days wear out of those. Umm, what else to try? Huge "granny panties" that utilize about a yard of white cotton fabric. Nope. Not comfortable. I cut the elastic out. They flapped too much and caused sensitivity issues. I tried oversized PJ bottoms that I cut to thigh high length, slung low like a bikini bottom so that nothing touched. Those worked if I stood still and kept my body in a vertical line. At the slightest bend, fabric would settle into a crevice somewhere that had to be pulled out, plucked out, squirmed out. That was a disappointing defeat. I KNEW those would work. What plan was I on now? Would I make it all the way to a Plan Z? One day I decided it didn't matter what I wore under my dress. Going commando. Even saying it aloud sounds powerful and confident.

I needed more long dresses and located gorgeous, cultural, hippie style, and beautiful skirts and dresses at the local thrift store for $3.99 – $4.99 per piece. What a win/win with my body covered and giving to charity simultaneously. Many complimented my new clothes, envious of where I shopped and how creative my new dresses and long skirts were. I smiled and offered a genuine "Thank You." Nothing more. That was my business.

20
MEET ME ON AUGUST 1st

Luke surprised me with a letter on our thirty sixth anniversary I will treasure forever. He seriously doesn't need to ever give me another card. This one is perfect.

"Here's the thing... 36 years is a long time in anybody's book. We have shared great joys and significant challenges. Whatever may lie ahead, we will deal with together. YOU ARE NOT ALONE! No matter what happens, always know I am on your side. I am here and will do whatever is necessary to make your life a bit easier. It is the least I can do.

We may have another 25 years together. I want those days to be as joyful and pleasant for you as possible. I want you to know ... I want our children to know ... I want our grandchildren to know you are priority number one in my life. You are indispensable. No one, and I mean no one, can replace or duplicate what you do, what you add, how you manage life for us. You may get a little slower as time goes along (as I already am), but know for certain this husband needs you and will make sure you have the best. I cannot begin to guess what our future looks like, not to even mention the next year. But know this, I am on your side!

I know your health is painful. I also know you are far better than you were two months ago. It may take a full year or more, but I know you are tough enough to do what you need to do to stay on the road of recovery. All I ask is that you let me into your issues. I need to be told what you need. I am not stupid or insensitive. I am aware of your pain and moods.

I cannot guess. I cannot read your mind or assume your feelings. You will need to tell me. I will do what needs to be done, it does not matter if it is convenient or not. This is not a marriage of convenience! We have a relationship of unconditional and unshakeable commitment. We will not handle our personal concerns alone! We will share them.

You are still a hot babe in my eyes.

Here's to celebrating our 50th anniversary in 14 years. All this is written with every ounce of love in my heart. You are still the rose of my life."

Random Thought:

My husband and I are closer in spite of lack of intercourse.

21
MEET ME IN THE ART STUDIO

With more time at home, recuperating and relaxing and trying to avoid stress, reduce car drives, and uncomfortable sitting arrangements, I had to come up with a plan. It might sound strange, but we only have one networked smart TV in our home. The insignificant, outdated black box style TV equipped to keep the children occupied with old VHS tapes was in a small bedroom. I had outgrown television several years ago, if that is possible. I was busy and rarely saw a program I wanted to watch. I know this sounds un-American but I wasn't into TV anymore. What to do with my free time? I could not read books as they did not hold my attention now. I had turned housekeeping chores over to my husband if they involved bending, pushing or pulling. I needed a hobby so I put together some ideas off Pinterest that seemed doable.

One of the things I enjoyed most was collecting nature objects from outdoors and creating collages. I visited a hobby store and purchased several sizes of blank canvases. Truthfully, that was my only expense and they were on sale. I used various color paints and tints from our garage, and as they dried, I planned the next step. Onto the blank canvases, now colored and textured with paint, twigs, dried flowers, intriguing shells, appealing rocks and varieties of weeds were hot glued into a systematic and creative/artsy fashion. Waa la la – I had become an artist!

Finding beauty outdoors and bringing it inside to be admired and shared throughout the year was satisfying to me. I gave a few canvases away, placed some in my home, and looked for other opportunities to share my primitive talents with others. One of the more unusual canvases I created involved collecting objects from various homes in which my parents had lived. Three homes were within driving distance. (Yes, I sneakily drove to two of the locations and quickly clipped a dangling partical of hedge, scoured for beautifully formed leaves, and plucked a stray weed or two. I contacted my brother and he gathered pecans, twigs, and leaves from the university my father had attended after marriage. His daughter was also summoned to the family project. She thoughtfully went to the dormitory still in use in which my mother resided and selected nature objects and included a dried rose. On that sacred block where my mom had lived was also the place my father proposed to her. This meant a great deal to me to have these various and meaningful pieces collected for the project. Finally, because as a child we enjoyed weekly summer vacations at Padre Island near Corpus Christi, Texas, I added a seashell to commemorate those incredible vacations. It was a random shell that one might find on a beach while roaming along the ebb and flow of the waves.

By creating family treasures, I felt like I was not wasting my time while trying to get "well." There was no time limit for this season of pain I was in. I did not want to look back years later and not have anything positive with which to remember this year. I had no art studio. I had a kitchen table but I felt like an artist and that is what mattered. My collage pieces were lasting tributes to life filled with purpose even on days when it seemed like a long day had no real value. Creativity was my answer.

22
MEET ME BETWEEN THE SHEETS

My body apparently has been preparing for this onslaught. My right hip joint was getting tighter. I had entered, gone through, and was on the other side of menopause. My calf muscles were tight most mornings and I walked stiff legged to the bathroom. I had stress – mind you it wasn't primarily my own generated stress, but I carried many burdens for others. One situation had left me frustrated beyond belief and there was nothing I could do about it.

However, for the most part I woke up happy, felt blessed, and was busy. My life was on track with creating a motivationally driven life. I enjoyed exercise. I ate the right foods. I drank water instead of soda. I slept 7-8 hours per night. I was rarely sick – as it was I had 119 days of accumulated sick leave. I was pretty darn healthy, inside and out.

My sex drive was moderately diminished but I attributed it to several things and it didn't bother me a great deal. Due to my hip inflexibility, I held my right thigh steady during intercourse. That seemed a little strange but who do you ask if this is acceptable or not?

But after February 7th, sex was THE LAST thing on my mind. Sex was not the instigator of this problem, but it was my final activity before I closed my eyes that evening. We set this aspect of our marriage aside and both of us concentrated on me getting better. We did keep in touch, literally, with manual massage techniques to keep the fires burning on my husband's end but it wasn't the same, as he would lament occasionally. He missed me.

As the months wore on, Luke began to ruminate whether we would ever have anywhere near a semi-normal sex life again. I, on the other hand, just tried to ignore the idea. In late October, Olivia and I discussed the issue. Ladies in my predicament had gone years without sexual intercourse, which made it even harder to resume once their bodies started to cooperate. The reason for this was that some women have waited years and tried to manage on their own without medical intervention. Therefore, Olivia felt less than a year without sex was still quite attainable and gave me a few recommendations.

One might suspect it would seem awkward to gain pointers, especially a woman who had given birth to three adult children! Au contraire! I was all ears; truthfully, the act scared the pants off me. I mentally processed her informative guidance for several weeks without discussing it with Luke.

At our next physical therapy session, Olivia and I discussed again how to resume a sexual relationship, specifically intercourse. This time she gave more clear-cut directives, and then motivated me even further by stating since I would be seeing the specialized OBGYN in ten days, it would be helpful for Dr. E to know where my body stood in the sexual area of activity. I agreed with her but was neither cautiously optimistic nor terrified. The adequate term was more like "reluctantly proceeding with the assignment in hopes it goes well." More days went by. I bought the "slick" lubricant, and began giving myself pep talks.

One late afternoon, I was feeling better than usual and shared this surprising information with my husband, that it was time for us to "try." I caught him off guard and he expressed deep concern he was going to injure me or, at best, set me backwards in the gains I had made. I assured him this was doctor prescribed sex and I had tools to make this more comfortable for me. First, I would drink a glass of wine. We would use lots of lubricant on him as well as inject it up inside of me with a children's medicine syringe. We would take our time. It would be permissible to stop and assess, and I would prop my hips up on pillows which would help relieve pressure. Olivia stressed this was about me and not about him. My deadline was coming up soon and I wanted to be able to share with Dr. E that I had been victorious with my homework. Luke processed this information and asked a few questions to clarify matters. "Okay," he finally said and we proceeded to give it a try. As it was, I felt we satisfactorily earned a B+ that first time and it was well worth celebrating.

From then on, Luke and I continued this activity on the days I had a massage. My husband could look forward to that and I could continue to amaze myself weekly that I was still a functioning female who had working parts that would cooperate. We did discover along the path that lying in the spoon position was easier on my right hip. Having a second glass of wine was not such a good idea though. Along with the muscle relaxers, the two combined gave me a migraine the next day, but this was pennies in the sea comparatively speaking.

This entire experience has opened my eyes up to the intricate systems of the human body, how precisely our pH balance, hormones, skeletal system, muscles and connective tissues, and primary organs all must work in perfect sync to achieve optimal health. I'm sorry I never took this into consideration and was negligent in my thankfulness for a sound body prior to 2016. I will not take you for granted again, my body, myself.

Random Thought:

Don't be afraid to say 'yes'.

23
MEET ME USING POWER WORDS

"**S**tudents, when you begin to research your topic, use Power Words. Instead of typing the word "animal," type "elephant." Be specific and narrow your search by using Power Words and phrases. Here's an example for researching elephants: elephant and diet, elephant and extinction, elephant and zoo, etc. Do you see how this works? The more words the better! You will find more information that will relate to your topic if you use Power Words."

I like the idea of Power Words. Yes, I could have instructed my students with phrases like "more defined searching tools" or "define your topic" or "research strategy." Too wordy. Let's use Power Words – Power to the People!

My Power Words from A–Z this past year.

Abductor muscles

Acupuncture and pelvic pain

Allodynia

Burning in vagina from diazepam

Can I sing with pelvic floor spasms

Can you stick a diazepam in your rectum

Chair cushions and pelvic pain

Commando

Constipation and pelvic floor dysfunction

Curing tailbone pain

Cymbalta and nerve pain

Directions for building an indoor hammock

Dry brushing

Fascia and massage tools

Fibromyalgia and pain

Hip dysplasia

Hip dysplasia and pelvic floor pain

Hormones and pelvic pain

Hospitals with therapy pool near me

Hotels with hot tub near me

How do you say fascia

How much Epsom salt do you put in a sitz bath

How to exercise your arms without using your abdomen

Hyro Massage at a fitness center

Hyperesthesia definition

IT Band and where is it

Massage tools

Magnesium and muscle cramps

Medicinal marijuana and pelvic pain

Nerve block

Oxalate diet

Paresthesia

Pelvic pain and panties

Pelvic Pain clinics

Perineal pain

Physical Therapy for Pelvic Pain

Pillow and pelvic floor dysfunction

Prempro dosages

Protein bars and 20 grams of protein or more

Pudendal nerve

Restorative yoga poses

Rheumatoid arthritis and symptoms

Saddle area pain

Sensitivity to underwear

Sex and pelvic floor dysfunction

Shock absorbers for car

SI Joint

Smoothie recipes

Treatment for neuropathy

Therawand and how to use

Vagina dryness and lubricant

Vibration in car and pain and cushions

Vulvadynia and cures

What do you do at a pelvic floor clinic

What does atrophy of labia look like

What is prolotherapy

What is an oxalate

What is estrodial

Where is the perineal

Yoga and pelvic pain

Yogurt and vaginal infection

24

MEET ME ON THE TRACK

A new friend was looking for a team of four who would help complete her personal mission of running several marathons. She would be using an online system in which teams tracked the miles they ran and hopefully came up with the number 2014, since that was the year of the online challenge. I told her I was interested BUT I was not an athlete nor a runner. I could walk, though. I could tally 30 miles a month if that would help. Without any hesitation, she looked me straight in the eye and said, "Yes, I would love to have you on my team!" We called ourselves the Sassy Sisters. The four sisters exercised on our own and not as a group; we emailed and texted each other to keep our spirits up and our motivation in check.

I did find myself longing to participate in a 5K. The fundraiser was 3.1 miles and there was no time limit for finishing. It wasn't a race but a challenge. I signed up for one and then another. As December 2014 closed out, I had completed three and was quite proud of the ribbons with medals that hung in my closet on a coat hanger. I am not a competitive person but earning the medals inspired me to want to join in on more 5Ks with like-minded individuals.

During 2015 I continued to find enjoyment by walking and jogging a little. When I say jogging a little, that's exactly what I meant. It may have been the equivalent of a city block but, hey, jogging is jogging. I enjoyed my gym membership, the city parks with walking tracks, and roaming throughout my neighborhood. I even took my tennis shoes with me when I visited my dad who lived out of town. There was a beautiful park with a walking track near his home and I liked to use it while there.

I had hopes for 2016, as well to continue my fitness goals. As one opportunity after another came and faded, I decided to compete in the 5K for the annual Cancer Center's fundraiser. I would enter regardless. I had known its founder, and this local labor of love was inspiring to hundreds as we recognized individuals who had been treated as a patient, we celebrated with those who remained cancer-free, and honored the individuals who had lost their war. The endeavor raised money for others in need of assistance while fighting their own personal battles with the dreaded disease. I had participated before but this year it was going to be a momentous challenge for me. I had signed up three months in advance thinking I would be strong enough by then to at least walk the designated route. When the day arrived, I wasn't quite ready for the full 3.1 miles so I revamped this challenge to meet my ability.

With excitement and anticipation, I went to the local training center and picked up my entry details with its designed T-shirt. I planned to walk the 5K in two installments at my own pace: one on a Saturday and the other on a Sunday afternoon at an obscure track. As I completed my final lap, I looked up and was astonished by what I saw. I was standing at an insignificant intersection and the street sign was labeled Victory. How had I missed that street sign all these years? I had lived in this community for over 30 years, pushed children on swings in the playground, fed the ducks, and enjoyed picnics in this secluded area countless times but not known I was standing so close to Victory. My eyes clouded and I felt accomplished.

Random Thought:

I have the desire to change. I will nourish my relationships to build possibilities and expand my vision. I will rely on divine power and wisdom. Love is a secret motivator.

25
MEET WITH A SMILE

If I hear "you look so tired" one more time or am asked "is everything okay" or am blatantly told "you look like you're ready for this day to be over," I will shoot myself. Of course, I won't. I don't own a gun – it's just an expression to show HOW FRUSTRATING this is! People who deeply care for you don't ask these questions. The others can and will say the stupidest things. So, I've developed a system.

R D S

Relax – close your eyes. Starting at the top of your head, release the muscles, around your forehead, your jaw, your neck shoulders, breathe out slowly. Let your arms hang limply. Feel your stomach go soft. Release anything that is clenching: buttocks, thighs, calves. Stand firm on two feet. Repeat from the top.

Drop - starting with your diaphragm, imagine a sinking towards your belly, going lower, lower, widening, a floating feeling - as if you were suspended in water. Do this a few times. Once doesn't cut it.

Smile - let your body know you are okay.

Random Thought:

I will take small actions to turn this journey around.

26
MEET ME AND MY PAIN SCALE

66 How's your pain today?" This is a frequent question from PT, medical doctors, chiropractors, and massage therapists. If you've not had chronic pain before, what do you say? You know 0 means no pain and 10 must mean you are about to end your life, but what do the numbers 1-9 mean? How does the written assessment of someone else relate to YOUR pain?

Pain is a part of life, the good life even. Feel the burn is supposed to be a good thing when exercising! You stub your toe and have a few moments of excruciating pain that dominate the senses. Some cry out curse words and others moan. Whatever your style is, pain hurts. But with rubbing it out, as they say, walking it off, you return to a normal function and it is forgotten. How does that kind of experience, which lasts five minutes, have any type of bearing on chronic pain?

When asked, I usually answered with numbers ranging from 2 to 6. But honestly, did the doctors and others understand what a level 5 was TO ME? Were they comparing me to someone else who stated their pain was at a level 5 but were smiling with no appearance of deep distress?

Olivia encouraged me to devise my own pain range based upon my experiences with pelvic pain.

0   Pain-free. I thoroughly enjoy this level 0 for about 3 minutes before I get out of bed.

1   In the bathroom, I start feeling the muscles pull in my right groin slightly. They are beginning to wake up. Reclining on a heating pad in bed, pillows under my calves and technology in my hand, I end many days with a level 1 ½.

2   Legs feel slightly achy as if I've pulled muscles while rock climbing. My legs feel like I am wearing leggings with plastic, scratchy thread running through the cotton which is irritating to my skin. I often check to see if ants are on me but they are not. I can sit in a chair for 15-20 minutes if busy.

3   This feels like surgery in my privates where I feel swollen and the sutures are starting to pull in opposite directions. Slight tugging; not ripping. A few horse-fly bites are now occurring in my legs and occasionally on my abdomen. I can sit in a chair for 10 minutes. I distinguish several knots under the skin – trigger points. My thighs and calves feel squished.

4   Horsefly bites now feel like bee stings on legs. Labia feels swollen like with infection and it hurts to the touch. Impossible to sit in a car for more than 10 minutes. My muscles running the insides of my thighs to the knees are painful. I massage them often. I will eat 1-2 meals a day because I know I need to.

5   Concentration is off. Go into a room and forget why I am there. Can't find things on my desk even though I just placed them there. Get lost in the parking lot at Walmart. Want to lay with a heating pad. Fall asleep in the clam shell position often. Use TENS unit for hours.

6   Cannot wear leggings. Force myself to smile. Now thighs ache tremendously. Walk slowly due to legs and abdomen. Feels like a minor volcano is brewing inside or else I'm in early stages of labor. No appetite. Hard to be around people.

My face looks like I'm having a migraine. Medication is not totally effective. I can perform simple tasks. Feels like my vagina and labia are beginning to rip. Cocoon myself in my hammock. Conversing with anyone is difficult for more than a few sentences. Reading and watching TV are not possible. Practice breathing techniques. I just try to get through the day in short increments.

7   Now I feel as if I am ripping out. Knife cuts in vagina. Mid-stages of labor in belly. Stay in bed with heating pad and total isolation. No talking at this point.

8   The only thoughts beside pain are my quality of life. I know I can't continue like this. I feel like I have been raped by a 2,000 pound gorilla with rips internally, externally, and a deep ache inside. I have felt like this twice – both in June of 2016.

9-10   I haven't experienced this level of pain in which suicide is an option.

Random Thought:

Please, please, please do not let this be hereditary.

27

MEET ME HANGING THE BLESSING BRANCH

It was a yard cleanup day. Blistery winds had come roaring through a few days before, which snapped dry limbs from their own family tree. Luke worked diligently by raking scattered limbs and twigs along with bagging fallen leaves which were saturated with rainwater. I put on a thick sweater and went outside to enjoy the cool, crisp air. An interesting detailed branch lay under an old tree which caught my eye with its curvatures that only nature can artfully create. After an ahhh-haaa moment, I gentled stooped over and dragged the lightweight branch towards the garage.

I carried the branch indoors and measured it and found it to be the exact size and proportion I needed. Peering into my craft supplies stowed in multiple drawers at the computer station, I selected a ball of yarn and six colors of felt squares. I trimmed the fabric into rectangles of various lengths and widths and placed these autumn strips of color into a beautiful crystal salad bowl. The four-foot branch was then hung with yarn over the kitchen bar that divided the kitchen from the dining room. This show-stopper was to become our Blessing Branch for the month of November.

Excitedly I notified the family of what I had created and enlisted their help. "When you experience a blessing, or are part of giving a blessing to others, let me know! I will tie a colorful felt ribbon onto the Blessing Branch for you, or you can come do it yourself."

Throughout the month, the Blessing Branch grew more unconventional with its colorful scrap ribbons. As guests entered the home, they couldn't help themselves and asked, "What is that?" With smiles, we explained the idea behind the Blessing Branch and many agreed they would like to start one in their own home, too. After all, the day of Thanksgiving was endorsed because of blessings shared. This project allowed us the opportunity to intentionally look for the good in each day, or try to. I so enjoyed receiving texts to tell me of blessings with requests to "tie a ribbon on for me." The blessing project was a tangible reminder of the possibility of good in each day, and we can learn to share in the blessings of others. It became a teaching tool for our little ones who were four and five years old. They, too began to seek out blessings in their own lives and enjoyed the object lesson immensely. This act of consciously seeking the good in each day and not putting much stock into worry about what might lie ahead was a tradition I may want to continue for years to come.

Random Thought:

"What we see depends mainly on what we look for." - John Lubbock

---

28
MEET ME INCLUDING
MY WALKING PARTNER

A lmost fifteen years ago, Bella Ruth (Ruthie) said she would like to ask a question. "Sure," I responded, "what is it?" Thinking she was going to ask me if I would help her in a task or bring a dish to a function, I was ready to help.

Instead she quietly responded, "I have been praying God will provide a walking partner. Your name came to mind and I'd like to ask if you are interested in walking together."

This caught me off guard. My thoughts were in rapid fire relay fashion, "You prayed for a walking partner? Who does this? And you feel God wants me to be your partner? Ought I accept? What if I don't? Do I have time to commit to this? How far are we going to go anyway?"

As you can clearly see, this was not an immediate yes in my heart, but I smiled and within a reasonable amount of time (30 seconds) told her, "I would be happy to become your walking partner! What did you have in mind? Where? When? Details please!"

We created a plan and it was easily carried out. Ruthie would pick me up about 2-3 times a week and we would walk three miles at a nearby track. Not only were we getting in great exercise but a deeper friendship unfolded. Ruthie had sons my children's ages and although she was a military wife, we had much in common as we discovered.

During the winter months, we continued to walk indoors and tried out exercise equipment at a huge fitness center in which she had access. I went as her guest. At no time had I exercised alongside a military soldier but it was enlightening and humiliating at the same time! They were in shape! Despite their physique, Ruthie and I continued our rituals and even began rounding them off with a sauna experience to sweat the world out of our bodies. I loved our time together and I loved her as well.

The military PCS's (Permanent Change of Station) soldiers and her husband were reassigned as predicted. I missed her. Ruthie moved to Arkansas, then New York, onto Texas, and upon her husband's retirement ended back in the state where we had first been introduced many years ago. Surprisingly for both of us, they settled into civilian life and bought a house only two miles from my parent's home.

We rekindled our friendship, long distance style this time. No weekly workouts or a walking track to use, but we would meet at each other's homes occasionally for catch up conversations about the joys and decisions we were making as middle-aged adults. Our children were growing up and having children of their own and there was so much to talk about.

I'll forever remember opening my cell phone on a Saturday morning in late June of 2016 and seeing all the condolences that were directed towards her husband on Facebook. I had this awful, weighted sensation that something horrible had occurred overnight while I slept. Within minutes I discovered the gravity of the situation. Their oldest son had been in a devastating one vehicle accident while on vacation the night before. Oh, my heart bled for her and the family. This could not be. He had such promise in the medical field, was the father of two, and the husband of an enduring young lady with many years to come.

I could not attend the funeral due to my body being in distress that day. I could not travel and it left me feeling empty. But as the summer evolved into fall, Ruthie and I made time for each other after my weekly PT appointments when I could. We once again became walking partners, as her body needed to move from emotional exhaustion and my body could not sit after traveling for the medical appointment. We both needed to walk and to heal. We walked slowly on sidewalks in her housing area. Her heart was crushed and bleeding and my physical body was ripping from the inside out. Together we walked, shared openly and honestly, and sought healing for each other and for ourselves.

Rounding a curve one late afternoon in a cul-de-sac, directly in our path was an enormous bean bag chair! It overtook half of the driveway, and it was set out for the trash. We examined it and found it to be in spectacular condition. Much to our surprise there were no rips, tears, or even any smears of dried food or yuck of any kind. We sat on it. We laid on it. One of us had to claim this freebie – you know "the treasure is in the eye of the beholder" type of gift. We returned to her house, found my keys for the SUV, and drove with purpose back to the cul-de-sac. The bean bag was still there! I lowered the back end and we casually tried to pick it up. Whew, this was heavier than it looked. We then began to heave and lift and then smash it into the back of my vehicle. I stayed on the outside, bracing it so it wouldn't fall back out – what little we had managed to shove in. Ruthie crawled inside to pull and I held it steady from the outside. It was like trying to ram a beach ball into a basketball hoop.

Laughter started bubbling up and we couldn't help ourselves – this was the craziest thing we had ever done and were the neighbors looking out their windows at the two of us on this impossible mission? How many others had tried the same rescue attempt for the now beloved suede bean bag chair we desperately wanted but could have cared less for just an hour before?

Jehovah Rapha – God is Your Healer. That day we had meditated in solitude and in conversation about how He was working in both of our lives as we sought deliverance from our afflictions. It was tough. But we also experienced the fundamental gift of tears of joy. God knows our need for balance.

In different ways, Ruthie and I were experiencing pain that felt it had no end and we were desperate. Nevertheless, as we walked through this season of life together, we grew and sought signs that God was with us. We tried to find areas of peace and places of joy that would bring life back into our somber lives on days that felt like dry, dusty roads of loneliness and pain.

We did not soar, we did not run, but we walked. "But those who trust in the LORD will find new strength. They will soar high on wings like eagles. They will run and not grow weary. They will walk and not faint." Isaiah 40:31

After all, we were walking partners. That's what partners do. We walk through life with one another.

Random Thought:

I want to live a life that matters.

29
MEET ME WITH ONE WORD

One of my Bon Temps sisters sent an enlightening and thought-provoking email during December of 2016. She had attended a class and learned a new outlet for making a New Year's Resolution. I must admit, I do love making a new resolution each year. I am one of the ones who doesn't just randomly pick "lose weight" or "be happier" or "clean out my closet" type of resolutions. I try to think them through.

When Lila asked us to examine the website "myoneword.org" I was intrigued and became convinced within a few minutes this was a place of substance and real concepts. As opposed to choosing a vice to release or an experience to try for the first time during the New Year, we were presented with the idea of selecting one word to center our life. A word that would bring special meaning and carry us through the next twelve months. A word that would be a work in progress, if you will, as you contemplated its description, nature, and outcome for your life. One word to provide a focal point. Others had posted on the website what the concept had meant to them from the previous year. Many had sought the guidance of how that word was found in scripture or in poetry, or simply in a dictionary or thesaurus. The premise was to select one word and hold onto it and not let it become lost like a given up resolution that didn't quite work out.

One word. One.

I could do this and I already knew what it was to be. Renew.

Meaning of renew: resume an activity after an interruption; to make something new, fresh or strong again; to begin again, especially with more force or enthusiasm; to increase the life of; to reestablish, revive, to make more vigorous, regeneration, reaffirm, replace, regain or recover, restore to a new or fresh condition, to replenish.

A noun, adjective and verb.
Similar words: adjust, alter, change and heal:
I WILL RENEW.

Renew my mind.

Renew my body.

Renew my heart.

Renew my relationships.

Renew my lifestyle.

Renew my devotion to my husband.

Renew my joy.

Renew my faith.

Renew my laughter.

One word with so many possibilities.

I can't wait to get started in 2017 with renewing myself – renewing my reality.

30
MEET ME AS I RENEW
MY REALITY

I had seen an art piece that inspired me to dig further until I was beyond amazed at the scientific principal behind the fragmented mural.
A turtle and a butterfly caught in the act of tear drinking.

Months earlier I had taken time one afternoon to color a page from
one of the new adult coloring books that were both popular and pro-
moted as art therapy. I believe in self-expression therapy activities so
I selected a black and white drawing of a turtle with a butterfly on its
back. As I chose my colors with intent from a modest stack of inexpen-
sive colored pencils, I realized this was me. I was the turtle. This was
my year to go slow, methodically, not win any kind of race, but put on
my armor of protection from the world and keep going forward towards
the finish line. Meanwhile, the colorful butterfly on its back was me,
too. This was going to be the new me that would be able to fly away
eventually from this desolate place called chronic pain.

One day I was reading a book filled with tidbits of knowledge, and
it briefly explained it is impossible for a butterfly to see its own beauty.
Its eyes are incapable of seeing its own majestically created and indi-
vidualistic wings that are designed for flight and life. Is it not true that
we ourselves do not see our own beauty?

I discovered a little-known fact: in Ecuador, a butterfly whose wings
will gently rest on the head of a turtle, will slowly sip its tears. The turtle stretches its aged head forward, almost as though to say, "Here, take

my tears. Let them be worth something." The scientific term is lachry-phagy (tear drinking), a method by which butterflies receive essential moisture and nutrients. Ama la Vida TV captured the moment and won the Wikimedia Picture of the Year Award in 2014.

This act of tear drinking with images captured on camera was phenomenal to me. What if I could use my experiences and lessons learned to help others?" I asked myself. "Can I do this? Am I stepping ahead of myself; will I recover?" The thoughts of turtles and butterflies fluttered in my mind as I played with various ideas. I am emotionally drawn to the image of the turtle and the butterfly. The butterfly is renewed from the sacrifice of tears. The turtle could withdraw, close its eyes and choose not to partake, but it doesn't. The turtle gives what it has for another. With sacrifice, another is renewed.

But be transformed by the renewing of your mind, so that you may prove what is the good, well-pleasing and perfect will of God. Romans 12:2 (World English Bible)

Random Thought:

I am committed to do what it takes to "renew my reality."

31

MEET ME ON MY BIRTHDAY

I look forward to the date December 10. Nestled in between Thanksgiving and Christmas, filled with anticipation of things to come: holiday party invitations, school break just around the corner, and December 10th, which is my birthday. Truthfully, how odd to be asked online for my date of birth when making flight arrangements and such. When given options, I scroll and scroll to find the year that matches mine. When did I become so old that I must scroll? Oh brother… You are as old as you feel and I felt pretty darn good… that was, until February 7, 2016. My husband often complimented me, saying when we were out that people asked if I was his daughter. I wore trendy clothes, had no wrinkles, and had a spunk in my step and a twinkle in my eye most of the time. I felt young. This age thing was for the birds.

However, this year I was at a loss. Leading up to my birthday I anticipated all kinds of horrible scenarios of what would become of me after this monumental birthday (the big Six Oh). Lord, when did that happen? But truthfully I had been aging in the last 10 months at rapid speed. Light speed compared to the previous year beforehand. I moved unhurried, I monitored what I ate, and I made no evening plans due to manifested pain and medication that sent me napping without warning. One minute I was sitting up awake, the next I was in a semi-coma. How many times would Luke come into the room and find me lying on a heating pad, mid-exercise but passed out from the medication that relaxed ALL of me? Two hours later I would emerge to discover I had missed preparing supper or a visit from the grandchildren who came over to play. Not a peep did I hear. I was in a new dimension of life.

Luke brought breakfast in bed to me on my birthday. You would have thought that started the day off in the right direction but all I did was worry instead; do I take my medication first? I mentally complained about the coffee with too much creamer and on it went throughout the day. Gripey, old me. Our daughter Christine, with whom I share a fondness for gardening, arranged to have FTD deliver an outstanding and beautiful green ivy arrangement with a 'Happy Birthday' balloon and box of gourmet chocolates attached. It was a thoughtful gift. I looked at the plant, and knowing how long ivy plants can survive even with neglect, underwatering and overwatering, I thought to myself, "This ivy plant is going to outlive me." My heart just wasn't in it. That afternoon I mustered up the courage to look happy. I pleasantly greeted family when they came over for cake, cards, and a few presents. I did appreciate their company. However, I simply wanted their company and not a birthday. I wanted to slide gently out of this year with as little ripple in the water as possible.

I had a hard time appreciating anything. Chronic pain was killing me and as much as I tried not to admit it, it was destroying my appreciation for those who meant the world to me. Thankfully the day ended with no big upsets and no one knew the inner me. But I knew who I was inside and wasn't pleased. Next year, I thought, you will have a "do over" and celebrate the life God has blessed you with. Kick up your heels and go all out, girl.

Random Thought:

Kool and the Gang have a great tune that plays in my memories: "Celebrate good times, come on!"

32
MEET ME IN THE GARDENS

I've embarked on a new tradition and that was to luxuriate in the tropical beauty with moist air while at the Botanical Gardens at least once during the winter season. INDOOR Botanical Gardens, I might add, as the temperature hovered in the low 20s. Since I can now drive to physical therapy appointments, I decided to give myself a well-deserved holiday. Before heading to the gardens, I selected a new restaurant I had admired. As we passed this ethnic restaurant each trip for physical therapy, I had secretly thought," I'd love to eat there." Luke is a meat and potatoes guy. He would have loved living on a ranch back in the day when made-from-scratch biscuits, platters of bacon and eggs, and canisters of brewed hot coffee were standards at breakfast, and the close of each day ended with savory steak and potatoes. Luke likes familiarity with food.

Christine had married a successful businessman who originated from South America. In fact, many in his family had now relocated and my daughter was loved and accepted into this new culture and loved it. The food, traditions, dancing, and celebrations suited her well. It seemed fitting I would drop in and try a plateful of authentic food before my next stop. It was delicious. Piled high and on several plates, it was way too much for one person at lunch but I enjoyed the pleasantness of the surroundings and the attentive staff. Eating out alone is not my forte. I can count on one hand the times I have ventured out to eat alone. Why do we so often assume a person who eats in a restaurant alone is lonely? Quite the contrary! I was on a mini-vacation with myself and celebrating!

Next stop was the indoor jungle. Its differentiated beauty with poinsettia plants placed in strategic locations as well as the focal point Christmas tree all worked in harmony to punctuate the glorious color scheme. I found a bench, got out my adaptive seating, and here was to be my station until physical therapy. I was in heaven.

It almost didn't happen.

Do you know when you have pelvic pain issues, it affects more than muscular pain?

"Like what?" you may ask.

What else is located inside the pelvic area? Yes, the bowel area and with the tightening and scrunching and pulling and tugging and nerve hypersensitivity in the general region, it was a given that a patient would have bowel issues occasionally. Imagine a kitchen drain under the sink. It will either be working well, or not.

Although I was blessed to find a parking spot nearby when I arrived at the Botanical Gardens, I was not blessed with a quick receptionist who was counting change and selling tickets. A leisurely pace, I might add. These deserving and admirable souls are volunteers so I shouldn't complain, but what she didn't know was that I had just minutes before I was about to have an accident. My Digestion Tea was working a little too well and I had a three-minute warning that day and, guess what, I didn't make the deadline. Thankfully, I was wearing long thermal type tights under my long dress with boots to keep warm. Into the restroom I fled and yanked off those tights while flopping onto the potty a little too late. It happens. It happens to all age groups but it is not socially acceptable to someone over the age of about four. After a quick but thorough clean up and with tights in the trash, I was composed and ready to enjoy the afternoon.

At times, life does not go as initially planned, and a girl just needs to get used to it. No one cared I was in the restroom for ten minutes nor knew I was no longer wearing tights or panties. Frankly no one cared. Life is to be lived, with or without accidents.

Random Thought:

Don't give up. You may be almost there. Why would you allow one more corner to stand in the way of your success?

33
MEET ME IN DECEMBER

When Book Fair time comes around, I get EXCITED! Just by selling the products, I earn new books, taken directly off the shelves at the close of the Book Fair and it's a win/win proposition. A stipulation is documented in the contract in order to receive 50% profit margin: sales must reach a minimum of $3,000. As the economy has deflated, the anxiety of "will I make it this year?" has increased. The final hurrah of whether we would see our goal attained or not was this evening. I had scheduled the Book Fair along with the annual holiday concert. Normally, this is no big deal but it was this year. Getting out in the evenings is almost obsolete, and with the temps at 40 degrees this evening, that tested my physical confidence as well. No shivering is allowed. None whatsoever. It only makes it worse. To be fully functioning at the school from 5:30 – 8 pm that evening, I took only half a dose of my muscle relaxer. This meant I would be in half agony as compared to full agony if I missed the dose.

As the evening unfolded, I realized I was going to make it through with no major flairs. I was not pain-free by any means, but I carried a smile on my face, was conversational with students and parents alike, and was able to operate the cash register and give out proper change. When you are "under the influence" basic math mistakes are a given.

A woman arrived whom I had not seen since July. She had visited our ladies' class but after a few months dropped out due to extended family issues hundreds of miles away. We hugged and I asked her why she was attending the concert at my school this evening. With great surprise, and did I sense a trace of indignation, she replied, "Don't you remember I told you this summer that my granddaughter would be attending this school?" I apologized for not remembering, that there were 800 students here, and I had not met her. She seemed perplexed.

What she did not know is I haven't remembered a lot of things. This past summer I had no confirmation I would be able to return to my career. My moments of pain were relentless; I felt knife blades inside my body and the clenching of muscle spasms seconds upon seconds. I had no appetite. However, I knew I must eat so I would place a piece of bread into the toaster, set it, walk out of the kitchen and not remember a thing. What a surprise to smell burning toast from the back of the house five minutes later. Oh yeah, that was me. I would start to sweep a tiled room in our house, forget the dust pan, and walk into the kitchen and then completely forget the broom, which was still in the other room. The pile of debris on the floor and the unattended dustpan still hanging on the hook would remain there all afternoon. Hours later, Luke would come home and find a pile of junk, and without questioning why, just take care of it.

My new friend, you have no idea what I have been through. My journey of how far I have come doesn't show. Forgive me, but it was not possible to have remembered your granddaughter was moving here and that she might be attending my school in the fall.

Random Thought:

Not knowing the future drives me to take one day at a time.

34
MEET ME FOLLOWING THE PARTY

L ast year's Christmas party was so much fun! Our school had not planned one in years, but due to a change in administration, which led to a higher feeling of optimism and overall morale, a party was in order. Not just a potluck, but decorations, games for the children, massive amounts of food, and Santa would be showing up. Just think, Santa after all these years, was coming to my school! The Hospitality Committee was thrust into action. After all, we were out of practice with pulling off such a huge endeavor of anticipated magnitude for ages 1 to 80. Yes, all family members were invited to come and to share the evening with one another.

It was a grand event and one not to be forgotten. I thoroughly enjoyed taking my two grandchildren who were 3 and 4 in age. Their eyes were wide with wonder and they uttered not a word when Santa arrived, true to life, out of a storybook they had read about but not once had seen up close and personal. Families hated saying goodnight but it was a school night after all, and we had to get home, bathe, and be prepared for the next day. A full class load of rambunctious students, who were also filled with holiday spirit, I might add, would be arriving at 7:45 am. We unashamedly enjoyed bidding those students farewell the next day for a full two weeks while we recuperated from one semester down; one to go.

A full year passed and the holiday season was upon us again. I had accepted a smaller role on the Hospitality Committee. My job was to send cards to faculty in the hospital and to those experiencing bereavement from the passing of precious family members. It was a solitary job that required little physical effort but meant a great deal to those on the receiving end. When asked if I would be helping to prepare this year's Christmas party, I politely replied I wouldn't be attending this year. How do you explain to someone half your age that by 4 pm you are in so much pain that all you can do is go home and stay there until the next day? No one at school knew this secret: intensive muscle relaxers, physical therapy out of town, weekly massages, chiropractic sessions to align my pelvis and hip areas, plus hours and hours of relaxation and my own physical therapy exercises allowed me no time for recreation. Recreation? I had forgotten what it meant.

Out of concern, the Hospitality chairman emailed me and asked if there was anything wrong or if there was something she could do. I thought about it for an hour. I admired her and could trust her with my secret but that would place a burden on her shoulders, the knowing of what I was going through. I decided against it and simply emailed back. "Thank you for your concern for me." She knew something was different but kindly sent back "L" – meaning Love. That's the best thing one can say when no words come. I was loved.

The one in charge of decorating for this year's party was new to my school. She had not seen pictures from last year, didn't know what was available to use for decorations, and was five month's pregnant and sick with a sinus infection. Therefore, with the help of several students the afternoon of the party, I started cutting the cherry red colored butcher paper for tables, laying out the greenery to run the length of each table, which would serve as a centerpiece, and gathered the many poinsettias plants and other décor that would add a festive and lively atmosphere to the 100 people on the guest list.

As the students came out of the holiday assembly at 3 pm that afternoon, they oooed and awwwed over the transformation from the basic cafeteria look to a Winter Wonderland over the course of one hour. I was satisfied and thankful we had pulled it off. I was a part of the party although I knew I would not be coming. Sometimes you don't physically have to be in attendance to enjoy the mood and atmosphere. I KNEW how excited the children would be seeing Santa. I could taste the wide array of many home cooked dishes brought to the potluck. I could see the smiles on the parents' faces as their children participated in the holiday games. I could feel the relaxation and the camaraderie between work associates as they set aside their 7-4 pm grueling job at times as a teacher, administrator, secretary, custodian, and other indispensable staff and came together as a family. I would not be there but, yet, I was. I had prepared the foundation and on that, the party was about to unfold in a few hours. I was part of the team. I did not miss the party; I enjoyed it in the comfort of my robe, my heating pad, and by viewing photos uploaded on Facebook as joyful friends came together for an evening of celebration. I was there in spirit and I was content.

Random Thought:

I'm living the life of about five people right now. I guess I'm a bit multi-polar. Me, me in pain, me in dementia mode, and me the medical researcher. Oh yes, now I'm a writer, too. I'm too much.

35

MEET ME AND THE
FAMILY LETTER

My family is in the undersized bracket. Both of my parents were "only children," so I had no aunts, uncles, or cousins. Rather than a detriment, I considered it a family blessing. We were close and enjoyed one another immensely.

It was now time to share the secret I had been hiding. I dismissed the convenient telephone call; questions might be asked in which I had no answers. So that my words would be composed well, I felt prompted to deliver my news via a family letter simultaneously. "Snail mail" style.

Dear family,

I have been dealing with a health issue and thought it would be an unnecessary worry to you if I shared it prematurely. However, this muscular dysfunction may be with me for a while more. I was recently diagnosed with pelvic floor dysfunction. My abdomen and pelvic muscles are tight and create spasms.

I have pain but am thankful I am now being seen by specialists. Please pray for me and Luke as this is a difficult season. I welcome any suggestions for relaxation that you might have. I would appreciate this information stay between us, as it is a private matter for me. With love to all.

Amy

My family "showed up." Liam sent musical downloads that would help relax the soul and body, my daughters both expressed concern with sensitivity, and my brothers sent encouraging texts without asking detailed questions. Dad candidly expressed he was there for me and I could share as much or as little as I needed.

It's times like these I am glad that I only needed to mail six letters.

How lucky I am

And how blessed I have been.

You're more than my family

You're also my friends.

36
MEET ME HALF FULL

The proverbial saying "a person either sees their glass half full or half empty" has been shared countless times. The content level is the same in each; it's the perception that changes. Do I see my glass half full or half empty?

Our holidays had been simplistic this year. No parties, fewer decorations, less time spent shopping, and so forth. We celebrated in our hearts more precisely than in outward expressions of activities and visible photos worthy of Instagram. On December 26th, I decided it was time to pack away Christmas. As I packed the greenery, inside mood lighting, and ceramic figurines into storage tubs, I couldn't help but become a bit teary eyed. Luke asked me a question unrelated to anything we were working on, and sensible me became choked up, grabbed a Kleenex and confessed I didn't know what was wrong; I just felt emotional. He didn't question me and thankfully didn't say a word. Even I didn't know what was troubling me that morning.

With realization, it hit me several hours later. I was at the six-month mark and my situation was not over. My hopes for an earlier, as opposed to later, recovery had come and gone, and my name wasn't on the A list. I wasn't on a list period, or so I felt. I was overwhelmed. The next morning was another day and I woke up to the question: Was I going to see this situation as an opportunity to improve and congratulate myself for making it to the halfway mark successfully, or would I berate myself since I was only at the halfway mark and had six more long months to go? Even then there was not a guarantee I would recover in 12 months.

It had been an estimation. But I like to meet deadlines and meet them early so this took a great deal of self-talk.

Last June you didn't know if you could even go back to work

You made it to Christmas and the family time was excellent this holiday season.

You have good friends who continue to care for you.

You are not alone in this.

You are strong and you will not only survive this season, but you will be better for it.

The water level remained the same in my glass but that day I chose to see my glass half full.

Random Thought:

Don't give up on your dreams.

37
MEET ME ON NEW YEAR'S EVE

I t was interesting to see what my children did for New Year's Eve. The three embodied what we frequently did on various family occasions when they were younger and lived under one roof. Christine was with many friends in the home of a work associate. The ladies dressed in sparkly and dazzling party clothes and the men in new Christmas shirts with jeans. The couples stayed up late, laughed, and loved one another into the New Year.

Claire took her two young children out for fun and thrills. She videotaped each one taking a turn as they crouched in an inner tube, which slid the full length of a long ice, covered slide and landed in an ice arena. During the day, they went to the zoo and viewed spectacular animals. At night, the three watched fireworks and huddled together for warmth and with laughter. Brother joined in the fun of playing with 'big boys' in the hotel's indoor water park and splash pool area. The incredible surprise of sweet little Sissy's face said it all when she sat atop the Cinderella carriage and was drawn through the lighted and tinseled streets, alongside best friends: her mommy and brother.

Liam adores the beauty of the mountains that are an exceptional showcase towards the north. He takes great pride in his physical strength he has earned through diligence in working out and following through with a dedicated diet. Being able to ride long distances on a bike is not for the weak in body and spirit. Due to the unseasonable warmth of the day, his ride into the wilderness to enjoy the solitude and fortitude of the mountains that are older than the Rockies but have been worn with age was an invigorating experience. I am so proud of his accomplishments.

Luke once said, "We have three children: one of each." And we do. It has been a pleasure to watch them grow and learn. We are in a good place at this point. This New Year's Eve, Luke and I chose to stay indoors at home. I created shrimp alfredo that could rival any restaurant's recipe and topped it off with pecan pie. Pecans from our own tree, no less. We didn't stay up late, kiss at midnight, set off fireworks, or have friends over. It was the two of us and lights were out by 10:45 pm. Together time, a delicious meal, and a quiet tone with reflective conversation were the best components in ringing in a new year with peace.

Random Thought:

Let go of what you cannot control.

38
MEET ME AND MY LIST

Here's a bit of good news. Every day has at least one aspect of "good" in it. Seek and you shall find, so to speak. Today's list written at the close of the day:

1. I drove to work and although it is a short drive, I felt little pain this morning.

2. I turned ten sizeable monitors on for viewing the announcements through the intranet system. If I wasn't there to do this, who would have?

3. Our book club had 15 students who enjoyed making upcoming plans for National Poetry Day, the annual Book Swap, and Brownie Day. Several students had thought provoking reflections regarding books they had read this year; characterization, twisted plot, and of course their favorite series were springboards for lively debate.

4. My energetic and happy voice over the intercom surely inspired at least one person in our building of 850 faculty and students.

5. Four 8th grade girls were authenticated as true artists when I offered to purchase their beautiful art pieces that were on display. One of the girls invited her mother to see the art before the $10 transaction was made. We had an earnest conversation on the reason of my purchase: to showcase the four words that the Bon Temps sisterhood had chosen in our "myoneword.org" project.

Each sculpture was unique and incorporated one of our words: Joy, Renew, Unafraid, and Strong. The mother was proud of her daughter and there were several photos taken.

6. I was available in my office for several phone calls that came through.

7. I sorted out the miscellaneous papers strewn about in the Resource Room from hurried teachers.

8. Two prayer partners reached out to me this evening by text message. We had a meaningful conversation with affirmations of living through the struggles of life and knowing we are not alone.

9. On the porch with my feet propped up, my eyes closed, I relaxed to the sound of a bird calling out to whomever was listening. I was listening.

In remembering the passing of my mom whose five-year anniversary entrance into Heaven was today, my Dad shared the Hebrew word "Dayena" with me: "It is enough." Life had been good for my mom and it was enough. Often used at the close of prayers, "Dayena" has the various definitions of sufficiency, I am satisfied, your blessings are enough for me, my struggle or my life is enough, etc. My day wasn't as good as my pain level was high, but by making a list I see that it was enough. It was filled with goodness. "Dayena."

Random Thought:

Counterbalance the bad moments with good ones.

39
MEET ME AS A WAITRESS

I confess; I have tendencies to overdo. Olivia and Dr. Hannah often cautioned me to listen to my body and move and stretch, but use restraint; don't overdo my muscles. Why don't I trust them, all the time? Ah, but it feels SO GOOD to work out!

A physical therapist in observation and evaluation training assessed me. She outlined a few new exercises to use at home and I accepted the worksheet with gladness. On it she hand wrote the number of repetitions per pose I was to perform. I began my customary physical therapy after work the next evening, and then remembered, "Oh yeah! I have new exercises!" Rather than go track the diagrams down, I proceeded to exercise from memory.

I proceeded to stretch, hold and lift as I remembered the directives. Indeed, it felt healing and invigorating all at the same time. However, something began to happen within a few days afterward and it was not good. My hamstrings grew even tighter. The muscles in the pelvic area ached more. I sensed more knots under the skin. I searched in desperation for the exercise handout and discovered to my horror that I had overdone it, again. I had been instructed to twist, lift and hold for a total of three counts but had instead done twenty repetitions. Instead of holding the new poses for five seconds, I had held them up to a full minute. Last year similar exercises were part of my regular routine for slimming and strength training in my core and legs. I had no issues with them then. But that was then. This is now.

I was saddened and my body language conveyed dejection. Luke came through for me when I couldn't on my own.

"We are not going to dwell on this. We are going to do what we can do, break it into smaller increments, and go forward."

Armed with this mindset, he planned a breakfast for Claire and grandchildren Z and E. They came over the next day and with excitement saw the transformation of our dining room table into a restaurant arrangement. There were plates, napkins, and utensils laid out as well as a menu for each. A stylish centerpiece adorned the center of the table. I was the waitress and helped the little ones read and decide what selections they wanted for breakfast. With efficiency, I wrote down their orders using a pen and pad, and passed it onto the chef, Luke. Breakfast was delicious and big smiles with hugs for the chef and the waitress were our tips.

That Saturday morning changed our directional course, and we allowed this breakfast to become a memory maker with many more good things to come.

Random Thought:

Never speak badly about yourself.

40

MEET ME AS I CHANGE

I was delighted when Christine gave me a canvas of a cougar image in transition as a Christmas gift. My school has a cougar for its mascot, and I have been collecting cougars for years. I find this art deco piece with mosaic designs to be captivating. I posted a picture of it online to see what others saw in this new version of a cougar. Some of the reactions were "I see a beautiful mix; a fancy cougar; colors – lots of colors!" Others saw a beautiful mask; gorgeous eyes; and one of my favorite statements was that the beholder saw serenity. "Endless opportunities" was a phrase I found interesting as well as showing confidence and being diverse.

"Would you like to know what I see?"

I see a cougar who is emerging into a new being with visions and with evidences of becoming a cheetah, a leopard, and a jaguar. The best of four, so to speak. I see artistic beauty and concepts of growth with the green palm branches hidden within the ears. I see directness and a willingness to move forward with the wide but intent looking eyes. I see a patterned and well positioned blue cross between the eyes to identify itself with purpose. I see flowers on either side of the soft forehead that provide beauty. The long, white whiskers offer protection from the elements of danger. The pink nose is an identifying mark of health. The multi-colored rosettes are intentional designs but painted with freedom. This animal with its mosaic adornments is both unique and one of a kind. It has an outward glow and is set apart from its darkened background from whence it has come. This newer and better version now has the characteristics of a cheetah, a leopard, and a jaguar while still retaining its original cougar roots. Not only can it run faster, climb higher, and conquer its prey with ease, but it is also a powerful swimmer who is opportunistic in many situations. This new and improved version is capable.

Once a Cougar, always a Cougar? No, not me! This new version of myself on canvas is placed in my Hope and Recovery Room. From time to time, I gaze at this amazing animal and marvel at the possibilities which await me as I emerge into a new framework with intentional formation. Will I develop new components for my new lifestyle? Am I changing more inwardly or outwardly? Am I becoming a newly designed woman for a purpose?

I will give thanks to You because I have been so amazingly and wonderfully created.

Psalms 139: 13-14

41
MEET ME BY MY MEMORY LOSS

I opened our local newspaper in early January. There was an article detailing the important lives and achievements of celebrities and other individuals who had died during this past year. I read with interest. It was a lengthy article and filled with interesting biographical information. Some names were new to me but to my surprise, I recognized many who I had not known of their deaths.

I was astonished.

I remember Harper Lee's passing on February 19. At that point, I was into my 12th day of this new affliction and was still operating in "this will soon pass" mode. Nancy Reagan and Patty Duke had died in March, Merle Haggard in April, Muhammad Ali in June, Arnold Palmer in September and Janet Reno was buried in November. All these deaths were complete mysteries to me. How could I have missed knowing of these? Where was I? Ah yes, I know where I was: inside the cave called Survival. I do remember Prince passing in April. I didn't even have to read further to know it must have been during the one almost pain-free week I had towards the end of April. Yes, Prince passed away on April 21.

Chronic pain is a thief. It has stolen my memories.

42

MEET ME ON A DIVINE ENCOUNTER

L uke and I met one week after we both had finished college. He was recruited for the summer to work at a sizeable recreational center for school age children, which was partnered with a large-scale church. He was the rec guy, the artist in residence, the whistle blower for tag relay games, the lifeguard, and the bus driver.

Meanwhile, I returned home upon college graduation to live with my parents briefly while I completed out-of-state teaching applications. I was determined to land an elementary science teaching job in the exotic area of DFW (Dallas/Fort Worth, Texas). But in the meantime, I needed money so I substituted for two weeks as a secretary in a state away from my dream location. It was during that week I was introduced to a young, athletic man who frankly didn't interest me much. He had just purchased his first car and nonchalantly asked if I wanted to go for a ride in his new convertible. Sure, why not? I received no favorable vibes as he talked about this car incessantly. Oh well, nice looking guy no doubt, but a little weird.

Throughout the summer, I waited impatiently for a job opportunity. In due time, I decided the waiting game was over. I would accept a sixth-grade science teaching position in my home state and a close friend from college and I would share an apartment together. A few weeks after school had started I saw the good looking, but slightly obsessed with his car dude standing outside in the hallway before a Young Adult class started. Yes, I was back at church – might as well, since I was now going to make this metropolitan city my home a second time around. I had dropped the dream of living in Texas. Briefly. I invited him inside and we sat together in the two available seats on the second row. The leader encouraged us to attend a Labor Day weekend extravaganza in Santa Fe for literally thousands of singles all over the southwest. "I need a headcount of who is going," announced the speaker and about 80% of the group raised their hand. When asked by the leader if I could go, I reluctantly said no. I could not take off the Friday before Labor Day to start the drive of almost 600 miles. School would be in session. That would reflect poorly on my reputation as a rookie teacher to take a day off the first week of school!

The dude looked at me and said, "Well, I could drive."

Oh, back to the car, I thought. "Are you sure? We wouldn't be able to leave until at least 3 pm."

"I don't mind," he said and that was that.

Have you ever ridden in a two-seater convertible a day's journey and within inches of another human being? Well, you make friends quickly, and that we did. In fact, by the end of the weekend, we had decided to become a couple. What a serendipitous outcome to derive from a National Singles Weekend! Luke dropped me off at my apartment and drove directly to his girlfriend's house and broke up with her. I should have recognized the strong opinions of this guy; seriously, who arrives after 11 pm to terminate a relationship? I wasn't so quick to break up with my boyfriend who lived in the heart of Texas. After all, I wanted to make sure, and what did it hurt to be a little cautious?

Our relationship status changed that weekend in the dense surroundings at the base of the Rocky Mountains. After our first date chaperoned by thousands, Luke and I realized that we were meant to be; within two months we were engaged. Sixty days is quick but we were confident and have stayed sure all this time. Thirty-seven years later sure. How do you sum up your marriage in a few words? We have experienced just about everything with one another. We clearly meant it when we said in richer and in poorer, for better or for worse, and in sickness and in health. Those marriage vow phrases are serious and require a lifelong commitment, daily dedication at times, to get over and under the rough seasons that develop.

We are in a season. Luke is going through all this with me, in his own way. He suffers, he is quiet, he is accepting, he doesn't insist, he is sad. When I have an idea on something that may bring comfort, he doesn't hesitate to lend a hand and make it happen. I brought home a horse trough from a cattle and feed company one summer afternoon; Dr. Hannah thought soaking in water would be therapeutic. We had previously taken out our only bathtub and updated our second bathroom with a shower stall instead. I needed to float and one cannot float in a shower! Hubby was a little surprised but quickly got used to the idea of a mini hot tub next to the outdoor grill, covered with a clear shower curtain clamped in place to prevent insects and debris from blowing in. It simply became a part of the patio.

The toilet chair, oh my. Yes, Luke made one.

My favorite all-time gift of love has been the indoor hammock. In the fall as the days became cooler I realized I was becoming despondent. I knew how cold air could thrust the temperatures from 70 degrees to literally 45 overnight. I would lose my beloved space, my hammock which hung outdoors between two trees. It provided me the ultimate quiet place where I could relieve my stress trigger points, enjoy the birds, sit in a semi-reclining position without being in bed, read or fall asleep. It held me in the right position for relaxation. Right away we began researching indoor hammocks. Why yes, they were available for purchase but had a hefty price tag. With a little ingenuity, and the displacement of some furniture in a bedroom, within a week Luke had handcrafted an indoor hammock frame and stained it a rich mahogany color to match the other furniture. I gathered some accessories for the room that would provide a "spa-like" atmosphere and named the room my "Hope and Recovery Room."

I love this room. I love the art, the carefully selected crystal geodes, the wooden pieces crafted and spelled with words like Peace, Love, Family, Hope. Seashells are in a bowl on purpose. A hippie style wind catcher hangs from the ceiling as an ornament with a big heart and trinkets. A throw rug at the base of the hammock has the look and sensation of a big, white wooly polar bear. I snuggle in the hammock with a furry style throw that reminds me of nature and God's creation.

It's a shame, a real shame as we have gotten closer to retirement that this has interfered with our plans. Would there have been a better time? Certainly not in my 20s as a new bride. Not in my 30s when raising three children and having a home daycare. As our children continued to grow, we were busy with activities, sports, and school events. We were the "Kool-Aid" family; kids from the neighborhood were either in our house or in the yard.

I wouldn't have wanted to have this in my 40s when my new career was kicking off after a crammed two years of earning a master's degree. I wouldn't have wanted to have this in my 50s as we were helping to raise our two adorable grandchildren who lived either next door or stayed with us many days and evenings. I would have missed the highly anticipated destination wedding in Cancun had I acquired this seven months sooner. In retrospect, I guess this was the best time. A silver lining can usually be found in most instances but it requires digging for it with retrospective consideration. The key to any crisis or trauma that occurs within your life and home is not to lose sight of the end. Today is not the end. Life is a gift and my troubles and afflictions are not entirely who I am. I set aside sections most evenings now to review scriptures, wise words and quotations that help focus my mind on positive statements. I need daily reminders.

Learning lessons, using new coping tools, and lifting one another up during trials are not learned when life is going well. Our marriage was a solid one. But there was room for improvement. We didn't listen well to one another. We were too quick to respond. We had our own agendas. We didn't yell and scream (much) but there was tension and anger that floated up from churning water occasionally.

As the months wore on, we didn't have the energy to zap what good days we had together with unkind words or selfish motivations. It's hard to admit, but I wondered if I might be a more focus-driven woman in the aftermath of this? Will my faith be stronger? Will my prayers be more meaningful? Will I sense needs and thus show compassion to others more freely? Will my priorities be redirected or will I allow this to tug on me, isolate me, and be of no benefit to anyone in the end?

Well, if I am going to have a dysfunction of this magnitude, it better count for something!

Random Thought:

I have changed but has anyone noticed the new, inner me?

43

MEET ME AND THE
WORD COURAGE

I t takes courage to get out of bed. What will I encounter today? When will the pain set in? Will I be pain-free for ten minutes or will I have the luxury of going one hour before the pain starts in and tugs on me from the inside out, reminding me that I am, in disposed.

Surprisingly, I am well. I have not missed a single day at work due to cough, cold, fever, or even a sniffle. I have not had a sore throat. My ears are clear and I do not have headaches. Nausea is non-existent. My blood pressure stays at a steady low range. When I fill out forms at the doctor, I am the ultimate boring patient who cannot even check off a single box.

Am I well or am I sick? Dr. Hannah reassures me that I am healthy. My body, specifically my pelvic muscles, just have a mind of their own right now. I am too well to be considered sick and I am too sick to be considered well, and few know my secret. The secret is I can hardly get out of bed in the morning for the lack of courage.

It's a strange world to live in; health and chronic pain do not normally coexist together. This gray area is like fog; no one notices. I stand at the back of the room during meetings, ready to dim the lights for a presentation or answer an incoming phone call. That's me - the happy helper. No one misses me when I don't attend professional development meetings anymore. After all, we are busy and it is only natural a person will take a sick or emergency day occasionally. Possibly it appears I am needed at work that day instead of attending a conference that would have benefitted me. Collaborating with others across the career curriculum would be deemed a worthy day, but I simply can't go. It's okay to not be missed. By not attending events, no questions are answered with vague answers on my part.

No one misses me at the gym. It's a big place and I was an anonymous but faithful member for many years. No one questions why I am on Facebook more often; after all, social media is the way of the world. But to many in the chronic pain society, social media is our avenue of keeping our mind and spirit connected to people. We can participate in conversations and experience the excitement of others as they share their lives, freely and without hesitation on Facebook. I can keep up, respond back, encourage the ones who are having a melancholy day, and compliment all in my own timing. I can sit in my bed with a heating pad and in a reclining position with electronic pads sending pulses into my tense and rebellious muscles all while reading short vignettes from others as they share their world with me. Thank you, social media friends, for reminding me I am useful and for giving me an opportunity to provide purpose for my life when, in fact, I am home in bed while you're not. Shhhh, it's our secret.

Random Thought:

She distanced herself to save herself.

44
MEET ME BEHIND A SETBACK

Ugghhhhhhhhhhhh

AAAHHHHiiijila;sdjfl;asjkdfl;ajskld;fjaslkdjfl;

WELL CRAP

What did I do wrong?

Re-assess

Heating pad and more lying in bed

Sleep and meditation

Mentally and emotionally checked out

Think only of this day – only of this timeframe – only of this one thing

THINK THINK THINK THINK

Isolation

PAIN PAIN PAIN

Quieten. So hard.

Cleansing breath

This is not forever

REPEAT: THIS IS NOT FOREVER

Micro-steps walking out of this dark tunnel

See the light – go towards it

Determination and set jaw in place – I will keep walking out of this….
OF THIS. I'm not going to stay here

I think I can

I'm better than I was two weeks ago

Cautious

Smile again

I AM getting stronger

This was a good day

I had a better day Thank you, God.

Content

I am me again.

45
MEET ME WITH SENSATIONS

The six months are up and I officially have CPPD, or Chronic Pelvic Pain Dysfunction. What does this feel like? I did a bit of research and identify with two conditions; one is considered a chronic disorder (Fibromyalgia) and the other has been labeled a disease (Rheumatoid Arthritis in the hips).

Deep and dull aches that start in the muscles and radiate out to the joints. The top and sides of my hips are stiff and feel swollen and tight. The insides of my thighs that attach at the knees are pulled taut from muscles and tendons. Severe pain, stiffness, and feeling swollen through my obliques, hips, pelvis, and thighs is a disastrous combination. To look at my naked body you will detect nothing. My greatest area of discomfort is in my thighs, pelvic, and groin area. Loss of appetite and fatigue are real struggles. I have an acute sensitivity to drops in temperature. Loud noises now are unnerving and drive me away from places and events. My short-term memory has diminished and my concentration is slacking.

The burning sensation in the vagina dissipated to some degree. THANK GOD. I sincerely mean this. It was originally caused by vulvodynia and began to lessen in severity after four long months. In the wake of its departure, because the muscles had been clamped in sure terror and intense pain for months, CPPD has developed. I guess it's a good thing I didn't know what was coming. Too much information at once would have driven me over a cliff.

The pulling of the muscles, particularly on the right side of the labia are bad. As muscles clench and pull, they shorten towards the pubic bone and are compromised in the entire abdomen area. This tightness loops around from the front to my backside. I experience little firecracker bursts and have knots across the bikini line area that feel like squishy earthworms under the skin; these require deep massage. Olivia covers her mouth and turns her head to not show disrespect to me but we both burst out laughing when I report earthworms are now hiding under the skin. My descriptions are plain crazy, even for her ears. For months, I felt I was in stage one for delivery.

As the inner thigh muscles seize up, my legs feel heavier. The area on both sides of my knees are pulled from muscles and are sensitive to the touch. I make my way slowly as if my legs cannot support the heavy boots that I'm NOT wearing. Gravity has shifted in my body and I am "glued" to planet earth. I do not have a light body that can jump, skip, climb stairs easily, or even walk briskly. I can stroll.

I sense bee stings on the backs of my lower thighs when there are no bees. I perceive other bites, stinging sensations, and painful sensitivity at the bottom of my cheeks (buttocks) that show no bruises. I have detected knife cuts up inside my vagina. For months, I could not lay on my right side for more than a couple of minutes. If I did, inner muscles around the uterus were pinched and tugged. After about five months of this, this sensation began to occur on both sides. I learned to lay entirely on my back. I have days that feel like my vagina muscles are being pulled out. I look down and see nothing amiss. Sitting is hard. Sitting in a vibrating car is a nightmare.

Physical therapy at home is saving my life with the on point, targeted muscle regimes that I faithfully do once, twice or three times a day. My free time is my PT time. I learn new techniques from the professionals. Unfortunately, this comes at a high cost. Treatment sets patients back between 24 to 48 hours afterwards. It's as if the muscles and joints know they have been found out and they are now resizing up their options for ways to retaliate. I'm at a loss as to what to do sometimes: do I go or do I not? I can't win this battle by myself. I need Dr. Hannah and Olivia's knowledge and encouragement. Their gentle words of affirmation that I will get better, that I am improving, and that they love their patients give me inner strength to fight this battle. I need them because they are the ones who truly understand.

Olivia remarks, "You have been through so much." Her sentiment seeps into my mind and soul and gives me validation that this indeed is a war. I am strong because I have not caved under.

Random Thought:

Would it be useful to mark on my body each bee sting, deep ache, sensitive trigger point, and pulled muscle with a permanent marker? Is there a correlation that I am missing? Would I eventually be covered in black smudge marks?

46
MEET ME AND MR. BROWN

M r. Brown, aka bunny rabbit, lives in my backyard. He surely must have handed the torch of life to another bunny but, to me, he is the same: Mr. Brown. My mom loved wild bunnies and they often scampered and hopped in her backyard. It was she who named Mr. Brown, the bunny, and it stuck. Forty years later, Mr. Brown is part of my life just as any other fixture in the family.

My mother passed away almost five years ago so seeing Mr. Brown is comforting to me. He's a living, tangible creation that connects me to her with frequency. I feel calm, relaxed, and content when I see him alive and doing well in my world. Then Mr. Brown disappeared for two weeks and it was beginning to look like the fierce winter temperatures were not in favor for him. I refused to believe Mr. Brown was gone… permanently. "Just moved over into another, warmer backyard," I thought to myself.

Luke drove home from a PT visit this evening. The session itself was good and the trip up and back was not as painful today. We returned home at dusk. So why was I sad and despondent? My husband was my chauffeur today and although I contend it was difficult to hear and converse well from the front seat to the back, hardly a word was said.

I see a pattern that is not setting well. I envision he would prefer to be with friends. I am not convinced he likes me anymore. He is putting up with me since I am his responsibility. I have become his interrupter in life. I don't mean it but I momentarily presume ugly things. What is happening to me? I don't use these words. My coping mechanisms are shutting down; the wall is being built stone by stone and it's a broader wall than it was last month. I am the wall builder and I do not know how to stop. I want to be alone and daydream of leaving. Let's just call it a draw before it gets nasty. You go your way and I'll go mine. I am a problem that needs to be fixed. No one has all the right tools. No one.

Where am I? I have officially checked out in mind and body. You can usually find me on the floor in a carpeted room stretching or lying on a heating pad. Luke prudently turns his attention elsewhere as opposed to seeing me in a comparatively collapsed state. Is this love or is this pain? Does his heart break to see my body at war? He walks away before I can utter a response. This is not conversation. This is marriage maintenance at its worse. No smiles connect us with sweet memories or plans for the days ahead. I am no longer sexy. I am deteriorating. He is my protector but he cannot protect me from myself. My inner voice asks: "Do you even find me interesting anymore?" I am too ashamed to ask.

After an almost non-verbal ride home, I opened the door to the kitchen and stood at the window, gazing out with discouraging eyes and a heavy heart. A flash of movement caught my eye and, YES, Mr. Brown was back! He didn't look my way but hopped through the fallen leaves and within 30 seconds had squeezed through the wooden patio fence. Quickly he escaped out into the outer realm of the backyard.

That might have been a bunny sighting for most people but not for me. Mr. Brown was home! I heard my mom's soft voice: "I'm still here, honey. Give it time."

Thank you, momma. I needed both of you tonight.

47
MEET ME BY MY GRADE

"It's been six months since your initial visit with us." Olivia asked, "How do you see yourself now?"

I answered truthfully, "On bad days, I feel I have made no progress at all. On good days, I am beginning to see the light at the end of this dark tunnel. I know I am better but setbacks are emotionally draining on me. I feel like I am starting all over and December was a setback."

Olivia acknowledged my setback disparity and replied, "You might try to envision a setback as a squeeze ball that WILL rebound and inflate again rather than feeling like a crumbled flower. You are stronger than a flower and I do see improvement. You are walking more freely and your pain does not show in your face as it did so heavily six months ago. You are using more coping strategies with success and you can wear leggings now instead of men's boxing shorts."

She suggested I consider this journey in terms of a grading scale. This I could relate to since I had spent 24 years in education.

"I believe you are at a C right now." She went onto explain why and I listened intently.

I later contemplated this score. When I first visited the clinic, I was in the failing range. A big red F. The F range is from 0 – 59 so at what point was I six months ago? How many steps had I climbed? Was I a 20 on the F scale in June of 2016? If so, this was great news considering I had climbed from a 20 to a possible 70: a grand total of 50 points in six months. Or when I entered the clinic, was I more in the 50% range? If so, I had only climbed 20-25 points. "How far had I come?" I wanted to know. "Was this good or really good?"

As a student, I generally received As. In fact, I was in the top 5% of my high school's graduation academic standards. Never mind that I took many home economic classes instead of higher level mathematics classes! An A is an A, right? However, I had a rude awakening when I entered college and realized how far off the mark I was in certain areas. My freshman year I sweated blood and tears in several classes but obtained a sad C. It was discouraging but the experience turned me into a never-giver-upper. After that first year, I didn't receive another C in a class.

Cs have their place. They prove you participated and did the home-work but accomplished less than the full breadth of the course. You learned but did not retain enough for the test. You did not fail, but you didn't excel either.

In this new course of life, I fully earned this C no matter how many steps it took to get me to this point. I expect to earn an A by the time this lesson is complete. I aim to be top of my class, even if I am the only student in this course.

Random Thought:

Guess who has second degree burns on their bum from the heating pad? Apparently, others do too because the term "erytherma ab igne" is listed in my dictionary.

48
MEET ME AS A PATRON

It occurs to me to stock up on Dragon Cream. How much will I need for the upcoming year? Maybe a case? If I am going to live 30 more years, how many tubes will I need? Does this stuff expire? Will aides apply it when I'm in a nursing home? You know, planning ahead!

I could write to the company!

Dear Dragon:

Dear Makers of Dragon:

To Whom It May Concern:

I LOVE your product. It is remarkable and I use it several times a day. (sounds cliché)

Dragon Pain Relief Cream is truly making my life do-able. I have Pelvic Pain Dysfunction and the icy hot sensation relieves the pain in my pelvic area, inner thighs, buttocks, and calves. The burst of instant hotness that stings and cools is absolutely remarkable with these stupid muscles that are stretching, twisting, and knotting up. (TMI)

Hello Dragon Friends: If you ever need a poster child for your marvelous product, I'm your girl. (too bold)

To: Dragon in Korea: Do you know how awesome you are? Fondly, your sincere and needy friend in the USA. (too emotional)

Hello! Dragon Cream is fantastic and I use it daily. (Would they even read such a short letter?) But is there a way you could develop a scent-free version? It's a bit overpowering.

49
MEET ME BEYOND
A COMPROMISE

W hat am I willing to give up for the rest of my life to reduce further pain? At what level of pain can I live with? That about nails it.

I am quite okay with saying goodbye to snow and water skiing. I enjoyed those high adrenaline sports when I was younger and I have fond memories, but I can let go. The adrenaline rush from Zumba will recede. Climbing flights of stairs will be substituted with an elevator. Bye-bye rowing machines, trampolines, horseback riding, and bowling alleys. Traveling outside of the US again is a mild sacrifice. Due to my husband's business, we once enjoyed many fabulous trips on the company's expense account in return for attending business conferences and events. Hawaii; Orlando; Washington, D.C.; Jamaica; the Dominican Republic and my favorite of all was the Island of Atlantis in the Bahamas. Traveling and attending concerts and sporting events were woven into our marriage but we are now content to watch them from our living room on a TV screen. Eating in saves money and is healthier for us. Restaurants are still enjoyed but at 5 pm to miss the lines. I have settled into compromise.

Most of my activities have already been adapted to one degree or another. In my ladies' class I have a cushioned chair while the other members sit upon hard plastic chairs. I tried standing up for two sessions and leaned against the wall, but that felt isolating. When we go out of town, I now lay in the backseat with lots of pillows to cushion the ride. Instead of talking on trips, we listen to music to pass the time. I walk slower and on level ground. I float instead of swim. I lay at home as much as possible either in bed, on the couch, or on the floor. Instead of entertainment, I'm focused on regimes of physical therapy. Most books don't hold my attention any longer so I read passages from inspirational authors and the Bible. I have no time to waste on life's drama. I communicate with real friends; my circle of friendship is smaller but more meaningful. I eat for nourishment now. I limit what I can carry, push, and maneuver. This pertains to carrying groceries, doing housework, lifting a child onto my lap, or a hundred other things. I step away when stress creeps in. In reality, I was not usually a person overwhelmed by stress until now. I intentionally back away from people who talk too loud, deflect and redirect conversations that are becoming negative, and stay away from crowds. Noise drowns out peace. I close my eyes, breathe deeply, and focus on a beach when I cannot get out of my immediate surroundings. The noise then becomes the chatter one might experience in the beauty of a sandy destination. I imagine the familiar salty air and I listen for sea gulls. I cleanse my thoughts and escape with these mental mantras: "Let it go," "Just for today," and "One day at a time."

Random Thought:

I am ready to write the Epilogue but I can't yet. My story is not finished. I don't even know if I'm halfway through. How many pages are generally in a book? 300? 400? Oh gosh, I hope I do NOT write a Stephen King type book with 900 pages. That is way too far to go!

50
MEET ME AND MY VOICE

F ollowing each physical therapy evaluation, therapy session, and medical appointment with the specialists at the Pelvic Pain Clinic, I would receive a questionnaire by email. At first, I was eager to express my thoughts in hopes of providing valuable feedback. After five minutes, I close the email. It was too detailed. There were questions that had no bearing on my situation at all. I saw no place for valuable insight. I refused to participate. I voiced my concern at my next appointment by saying patients with chronic pain cannot complete the survey as it is long and complicated. Honestly, it just makes me upset when I try to fill it out.

Here's my insight:

Dr. Hannah has evaluated me and I have seen her several times for physical therapy since our initial 1 ½ hour session. I have appreciated her approach, techniques and compassion so very much. Her optimism keeps hope alive.

I traditionally see Olivia for physical therapy. Her explanations are understandable and yet in depth regarding my condition. She ensures that I have learned how to do PT at home successfully. She speaks to me in positive statements. She understands when I am having a bad day and does what she can to help subdue the pain. Both Dr. Hannah and Olivia are helping me to cope mentally and physically.

I would also like to show appreciation to the office staff as they greet me personally by name and truly see me, rather than a patient who comes in weekly.

This is what I cannot write on a survey since it doesn't ask.

Random Thought:

I'm bagging up all the clothes that I no longer wear. Pants for sure are going in the bag. Short skirts and dresses will be next; I can't risk someone seeing my white boxer shorts for men peeking out from under the hemline! Now I won't see all the negativity hanging in my closet.

51

MEET ME WITH THE HONEST-TO-GOD TRUTH

"GOD, I don't like to journal. I don't want to go to a therapist and explain everything that is going on with my body, spirit, career, faith, absence of goals, loss of who I am and what I expected to be. I don't want to go pay money to talk about the crap that has come into my life. Feb 6, 2016 was a fine enough day. I CANNOT FATHOM how I went to sleep and woke up completely changed. EVERYTHING HAS CHANGED. How can things change so much in your life, your total life, when you are peacefully asleep?

I'm perplexed, saddened, disappointed in me, and feel an incredible shortfall for the family because they have lost who they remember as their mom. I don't even want or can't even be around them sometimes. The expectations are overwhelming. The noise, the conversation. I'm so different; the real me. looks like I'm there but I'm now invisible. They don't know me. I disappoint everyone, including myself.

So, what's up? Why did I get picked for this? And how about the even smaller percentage of patients who aren't cured as predicted? I THINK THIS IS GOING TO BE ME! Why am I not going to get to enjoy life like normal people who are retiring and looking forward to new goals and opportunities for themselves, their families, new service projects? Meanwhile, it appears I will STILL BE ALONE IN THIS ROOM DOING HOURS OF PT every single day for the next year – simply in hopes the pain will go down 50%. HOPING. NO GUARANTEES. This is the most stupid predicament I have ever been placed in. EVER and I mean EVER EVER EVER EVER!!!!!!!!

I'm confused, sad, mad, hurting, and feel truly alone. I am supposed to know my body the best, they say – and it's a total mystery to me. I can't even plan for next month much less months and years from now. It makes no sense to make plans. I can't fathom living like this for the rest of my life.

I REALLY WOULD LIKE FOR YOU TO CURE ME. I know you did it in the Bible; those stories of people going into remission / submission for a while, maybe longer with things, but deep inside I don't know if this is for me. No security in anything anymore, except the promise of Heaven. Is that all to look forward to these days?

I can't combine, effectively, my inward terror and isolation and lack of control – all this – with the verses that I am reading to diminish fear. My feelings and the knowledge that YOU are in control are at war in me. I'm bipolar these days with humanness that is at its worst and meanwhile trying to rise above it all with absorption in scripture and positivity. My body is playing tug of war with my spirituality, my emotions, my thought patterns, and most definitely with my physical body, which HURTS ALL THE TIME. DOES ANYONE GET what it is like to HURT ALL THE TIME. FOR OVER A YEAR? How is this even possible?

My husband is filling out all my retirement information. I don't even care anymore. Retirement for me has turned into convalescence which is TOTALLY DIFFERENT than what I worked my butt off for with the school system for 24 years… for it to come to this.

I turned into a senior adult while I slept for 7 hours. A senior adult who is very senior adultish with their primary activities of going to doctors and church. That's it.

If this is the way it is going to be for the next 20 years, I cannot handle it. I MEAN I TRULY CANNOT HANDLE IT. I hope I just die in my sleep and get it over with rather than live like this for 20 years. What is the point?

My pain tolerance is high. I believe with all my being that when I say I am hurting at a pain level of 4 – anyone else would say it's a 5 or 6. I have endured way too much this year and I AM SICK OF IT.

SICK SICK SICK SICK SICCK OF ITTTTTTTTTT

There. This is why I don't want to go spend $75 talking to a thera-pist to get all this garbage out. It's filthy, spoiled, wasted time, hours and days that have piled up into a heaping pile of over 375 days so far and I have NO ANSWER.

This is the most honest and truthful prayer I will ever write. Only with true intervention will I make it. I'm begging, like laying on the floor holding onto your leg as you walk away from me, begging that you take this burden off my body and help me live well again. My faith is weak. My trust is low; I feel, somehow, I just don't matter enough in the whole scheme of things to have this one shrinking body fixed."

Random Thought:

Say exactly what you mean.

52
MEET ME IN THE RAINFOREST

If I could design the perfect physical therapy clinic for pelvic pain patients, I would choose a rainforest theme. Lush foliage would line the walls of the waiting area. Parrots and songbirds would be in beautiful cages and set the tone for peaceful surroundings. Glow lights made from salt mines would lighten darkened corners. Instead of reading magazines while waiting, ladies would be offered a headset upon arrival in which melodic rainforest harmonies would help subdue the mind and body. Chairs and soft comfy couches would beckon its guests with soft hues of green and in shades of blue – the colors of leaves and water.

Once called, ladies would enter the rainforest and their gaze would lift upward into a waterfall that cascades into a compact pool; koi fish would swim just under the surface. Sounds transmitted through audio technologies would imitate inhabitants, calling to one another. Sauna rooms would cleanse the body after a session. An exercise room would have screens on its equipment to recreate the ideal rainforest ambiance. At the end of the exercise room, a shallow pool with painted lanes would be available for strength training. Walls would be adorned in mosaic tiles, fabric drapery, bamboo screens or wooden adornments. Hammocks would hang from branches for those who wished to relax following a session. Peace would pervade.

The space would be identified as The Rainforest – a peaceful alternative for Pelvic Floor Physical Therapy. Close your eyes, can you sense it?

53
MEET ME WITH MY QUESTION

AM I HEALING? I don't know? AIIAIIAIGHHHHHHhhhhhhh!!!! I can't tell.

Mental checklist…

2/3 less muscle relaxers

No Diazepam in a month

The last time I used a heating pad for pain was after my PT appointment. That is to be expected. No cause for alarm.

I haven't lost my car in a parking lot in a few months.

I'm happier and laugh more often.

I look refreshed and have a healthy glow.

I can walk two miles at one time for exercise. I added in 250 jogging steps going downhill.

I can bend over and unload the dishwasher.

I poop freely.

The bee stings are leaving.

I can carry two gallons of milk at one time.

I prepared lunch and dinner almost every day this week.

Wait, I just got a bee sting in my left calf. This is the tenth one RIGHT THERE today.

No napping this week.

I can remember items from a simple shopping list.

I'm using the heating pad again but that's okay.

I'm hungry and have gained five pounds.

Bad idea to jog. No more jogging. Legs too tight.

Loud noises do not startle me.

I'm tapering off medication.

My legs are not in toothpaste squish mode.

I sang aloud and it didn't set off abdomen spasms and tight muscles..

I was happy today.

I forgot to place my suitcase into the back of the car. My clothes are still back at the cabin, in the driveway, three hours away.

Seatbelts are still uncomfortable. No, they are unbearable.

I feel a band of tight muscles cinching me up.

Panties are out of the question.

Bee stings have returned. What does this mean?

I left the house and ran six errands.

I can't wait to get home and jerk these panties off.

I'm not ready to taper off medication.

I had a social at my house last week.

I don't believe my husband would mind if I wear his briefs.

I believe I am getting better.

Random Thought:

I received a letter from my insurance company with these words in big bold print: WHAT HAS CHANGED IN YOUR LIFE? I burst out laughing!

54
MEET ME AND THE GIFT

As we passed one another in the front office, I greeted my friend Liora with a customary "Good morning." We stopped to chat for a few minutes before the hustle and the bustle would erupt at precisely 7:45 am – bus arrivals with hundreds of energetic students. We two were early birds and liked it that way. Sipping our coffee and catching up from the day before, I noticed a stunning beaded necklace hanging around her neck. I commented, "That is so beautiful. What a unique beaded cross."

She smiled, "This is one of my favorite pieces and it goes with just almost everything. I think it looks Old English, like it came from a castle or monastery."

I agreed, and with a smile and a twinkle I asked her, "Will you leave it for me in your will?"

Liora is younger than I, so this was an improbable situation and she knew it, but she laughingly said, "Of course I will!"

I discovered later Liora continued to think about my request. She was one of the three who knew a little of my predicament this year: I simply had a health issue involving pain and nerves and that this would be my final year in education. True to her word, she had kept the secret and I appreciated that. But it did give her a new level of understanding regarding the challenges I faced.

Around noon, I walked across the hall and into the office to retrieve my mail that had been delivered. Opening my teacher box, I gazed at the beaded cross necklace. A card was attached and it read: "Sweet Friend. You asked me to leave the necklace to you but I can't wait that long. I want you to have it now. I insist. With Love, Liora"

"Thank you for the necklace. I will cherish it. You are a Gift to me, Liora. I love you I love you back." The aroma of lovely friends is heaven's scent.

Random Thought:

In a gentle way, you can shake the world. Mahatma Gandhi

55
MEET ME IN A POEM

Me

Who am I? I don't know

This thing is taking over.

I can't think, do, plan

I can't

BE

I can't be anymore.

It's too much for me. It's too much for

YOU.

What is Hope

Hope for me is slight

So very tiny

Buried under.

It's there

Look.

Micro sized

Dormant but waiting.

But it's there, nevertheless.

Hope never leaves

Hope never gives up

I must not forget.

Hope is below

Hope is an invisible foundation

Hope supports the weight.

Hope is strong.

Hope holds me up

Hope grows

Hope is beautiful

Hope gives power

Hope will save me.

Love and Pain

Pain and Love

Which is more

More?

Which is larger

Larger?

Which wins?

Wins?

Love always Wins.

I hate my Barbie legs

Can you see my seams?

Snap

Disposable legs

malfunctioning

Can I dispose of them?

Squeezing, throbbing, shocking, stabbing, biting, aching, pulling

PAIN

Unperceived, the enemy under the skin

Is pain real?

My Barbie legs are my division line

The invisible line of attachment

Tug of war

North and south

East and west

Who prevails?

Muscles pulling underneath the cover

of me

It feels that I am losing

My legs feel broken off

I am shattered

Separate isolated detached

And I am dying from the inside out.

Barbie legs

Sometimes I cry

Alone

I don't want to burden you

Nor carry the weight of your pity

And fear

So, I cry

Alone.

I cry for regret

I cry for tomorrow

I cry for loss

I cry with acceptance

I am losing myself

One day at a time

It will be a very slow process until

No pieces can be found of me at all.

I am healing!

Possibility or Impossibility?

Dare I dream?

Should I say the words aloud?

Will people look away due to their unbelief?

Not mine.

Will sweet sorrow show in their eyes?

Will they think I am unaware of their sentiments

that I am incurable

delusional

And childish

Will people notice that I am returning?

I am and I will.

Rest, Relaxation, Renewed

Returned, Rejoicing

The Sea calls my name

Come

Enjoy

Relax

At the Sea.

A time and space

For restoration

For healing

Power Beauty Reviving

Constant and sure

Alive

I am

The Sea in me

56
MEET ME DOWN TO MY TOES

M e to myself: "My face doesn't hurt. Nor my hair. My fingers are fine. My hands sometimes ache but that was going to happen anyway due to the fact that I have early stages of arthritis setting in. Therefore, let's not count the hands either. My elbows work great. My knees are okay – no popping. My ankles aren't swollen. My toes look and feel as I remember."

My Grandmommy endured the effects of polio from the age of eight on. Her feet remained twisted after she was released from polio's stronghold and soon began to wear orthodontic shoes. I still maintain that I inherited my body style and petite-sized feet from her. My shoe size is a size 6.5 and my toenails are hysterically tiny. It's almost useless to paint them as you can hardly find a toenail on "this little toe had roast beef" and pinky toe "this little toe had none." Nevertheless, it was time to celebrate the toes and the lack of pain in them. After a nice warm shower, I trimmed the nails and pushed back the cuticles to expose as much nail as possible.

I ask myself, "What color will I choose? A remarkable, memorable color!" I decide on purple. Of course, it's the sign of royalty so on went the purple nail polish with a final coat of glittery clear lacquer. Now when I look down in the shower and see my toes, I smile. They remind me that I'm still me, part of my beloved grandmother, and that I can experience wholeness in those parts of me that are vitally important. Focus on the good; not ALL OF ME is in distress. Toes matter.

57

MEET ME WITHOUT COMPLAINTS

P astor Will Bowen of Christ Church Unity in Kansas City, Missouri introduced a wildly, creative idea: the No-Complaining Bracelet. The hope is to get people to catch themselves complaining and switch modes into something more grateful. Their site "A Complaint-Free World" has several supportive ideals and tools to help make this a reality. The Bible has much to offer as insight regarding our words and thoughts. I believe God wants us to talk, cry, plead, share, and even express anger. But sometimes, don't we all get stuck with dwelling, obsessing and rolling on and on with our complaints to anyone who will listen? What I hope to gain by wearing the bracelet is to review my words (vocal, written, and inwardly) and turn them into short but truthful statements and positive comments instead. Complaining generates regret and unhappiness on my end, and pity and sorrow from others. I have chosen to wear a favorite bracelet and practice the same concepts of switching the bracelet to the other wrist when I slip and voice a complaint. This will allow me to critique myself and then hopefully do something about it.

Admittance: The first item listed in the Alcoholics Anonymous 12 Step Program.

Almost 11 months into this chronic pain issue, I have complained aloud, cried, screamed, isolated myself, journaled, redirected, laid down, stood up, prayed, massaged, under medicated, over medicated, slept, slept fitfully, and done everything possible to alleviate my pain and get 2016 behind me. I have complained to myself, to my husband, and to God. I have stated facts when asked. But in earnestness, given the severity of this condition, I am convinced I have not overdone it. However, the year has come and gone and I have a fresh start to do better. I will strive not to complain about simple issues that arise from daily life.

Chronic pain is severe and is a whole different category of life. But I will choose to not complain even if this lasts another six months. I'm hopeful for a miracle but I won't complain if it doesn't happen. Worse things are out there.

Random Thought:

The Lord gives His people strength. The Lord blesses them with peace. Psalm 29:11

58
MEET ME ON THE RUNWAY

" Are you doing any type of cardio exercise?" Dr. Hannah asked. Sadly, I admitted, "No." My last cardio had been during the first week of May. Now that had been fun! The local community hospital had partnered with our middle school and an elementary feeder school to conduct a fitness activity. Fifty or so students from my school were selected with several sponsors and we walked with the incoming 6th graders back to their school after they arrived at ours. It was an all morning affair to include students from both schools walking each way. Our school would then hosted fun activities to motivate these new students regarding how exciting next year could be for them. Of course, snacks were provided during the intermission. I was on the welcoming committee and as students entered the building, we guided them to many indoor events. It was a fun morning which totaled up to three miles in distance.

I prepared for the event by wearing a low slung skort that was soft cotton so that precious body parts wouldn't rub. I wore sound tennis shoes. I had an upbeat attitude and enjoyed this Fitness for Health event immensely. As a surprise bonus, I connected with a friend who now worked as a fitness coordinator for the hospital who organized the event and participated as well. It was a fun day! Unfortunately, that was the last fitness event I remember doing the remainder of the year.

As months wore on, my body just couldn't keep up; I slowed down. I did not stride; I strolled. When I could not stroll, I shuffled. By December I was one big mess and when the question of cardio came up, I gave myself a thumbs-down, but what could I do? I was not a member of a gym that had a warm indoor pool. I wanted to get back to walking, but how? Mummied up with a full parka because my internal body temperature seemed to have dropped during this period of inactivity, I set out to stroll a few blocks on a marginally warm day. To my surprise, I discovered if I intentionally swayed my hips back and forth (unseen beneath the huge parka) I was able to move a little easier and go a tad faster. The next day and the next I practiced on my experiential gait. This was not a waddle; I was now a model, walking the runway. If I swayed but held my head up high, it seemed to relax my front abdominal muscle group. Without swaying, the abdomen would begin to tense up again as I held my head up and began to suck it in.

In this new phase of life, sucking it in is not an option. Instead, we are instructed to let it all hang out. By the fourth day of this new form of walking, I had more freedom to pick up my feet without the weight of a heavy, internal object bearing weight on my hips all the way to the soles of my tennis shoes.

Talk about a light bulb moment that changed the course of my recovery; this was it. Sway those hips, girl! Instead of hiding my tennis shoes in the closet, inactive and forgotten, I placed them in the bathroom as a visual reminder to use them and enjoy the new freedom they brought back. I told myself "You got Sway, girl!" and I allowed my mind to believe I indeed had style, personality, and inner power. The way you carry yourself says a lot.

59

MEET ME IN DESTIN

" The cure for anything is saltwater – sweat, tears, or the sea." - Isak Dinesen

I'm a sun worshipper. I love the heat in the summer. I adore summer clothes. I enjoy getting pedicures to show off stylish sandals. The long days from sunup to sundown which last 15 hours are my favorite. I've been to beaches in Texas, Florida, California, Mississippi, Louisiana, North Carolina, Ixtapa Mexico, and Cancun. Due to an unexpected but interesting job opportunity for Luke in December of 2007, we traveled on a business expense account to exotic beaches. Mind you, these were annual conferences but there were big slices of time each day we were left on our own to explore and soak up the surroundings. With the convenience of an airline ticket, we went from the plain and ordinary to basking under the palm tree called "the rich and famous"… or so we felt like it anyway. During those years, we delighted in the surf and sand in Jamaica, the Dominican Republic, Hawaii, the bay at Epcot and Disney World, and best of all on the island of Atlantis in the Bahamas. Oh my, if I could afford it, I would drop all plans and venture back to this oasis of wildlife, beauty, and sanctuary on a yearly basis. Atlantis was the dream of all dreams.

I have a new dream. It's not a world vision dream worthy of a speech, a book, or even a video. My dream is close and personal and I can't quite put into words what the reality of it coming true holds for me. My dream is to visit Destin, Florida during the summer of 2017 as a celebration of three important events in my life: Turning 60 years of age, retirement from public education, and the grand finale to the ending of this Pelvic Floor Muscle Dysfunction. I have planned my entire life to keep my body fit. If you eat well and exercise consistently, a person can stay trim and attractive throughout life. I will wear a bikini on the Emerald Coast at Destin.

I envision the waves. I feel the sand beneath my exposed toes. I relish the saltwater bath on my body. I look forward to receiving a brief sunburn due to overexposure. I want to see sea gulls again and throw bread into the air and watch them devour it. I can sense the peace, quiet, and calm only a beach provides.

I have seen designed pieces to wear as jewelry which hold a beloved one's ashes; these are artistically created to be worn as a covenant between you and that person. A timepiece set in silver or gold that identifies you are forever with the loved one. I will purchase one filled with sand I have sifted through and gently poured in from the Emerald Coast in Destin. I want to feel the sustaining power this beach will provide, hanging around my neck. I haven't even gone yet but I want, and need, a permanent reminder of this celebration in Destin.

Time will not be a problem. Money has been set aside. I am doing everything I can to prepare my body for the release of this phantom. I pray He will honor my request and allow us to go.

60
MEET ME IN THE FIRE AND THE RAIN

I am partial to music from the 70s and can relate to many of the melancholy lyrics at this point in life. I intently listened this week to lyrics from James Taylor's "Fire and Rain." A mid-portion of the song resonated with me and since I was alone in the house, I began to free dance, steadily moving to the beat as my body, mind and soul became one.

Indeed James, I, too thought my sunny days would go on. I've felt lonely and reckoned my days were without end. Calling aloud to the only one who can help is the sole way to make it on this road with no end. A journey sealed with desolation and pain. Your loss comes from losing Susannah; my grief comes from losing myself.

I thought I would see ME again. Will I?

Unashamedly the tears flowed down my face and dripped off my chin. But I continued to dance. It's too early to give up but I believe James would not mind if I mourned. I have gained and I have lost. I am treading water.

61
MEET ME BUT WHO AM I?

Mother, Daughter, Friend

Problem Solver, Doer, Planner, Organizer

Worker Bee

Enthusiastic, Motivator, Encourager

Determined

Writer and Reader, and a Poet when inspiration strikes

Observant, Listener, a Well-wisher

The Ultimate cheerleader

Plan B, that's me

I am drawn to art

I try new things

I'm still Me inside!

Hello me. You are not forgotten.

62
MEET ME WITH A MISTAKE

W hatever you do, don't pick up the Dragon Pain Relieving Crème, squirt a sizeable amount onto your toothbrush and proceed in the morning drill of brushing your teeth. This might happen next:

Thoughts in rapid fire motion…

This is a really strong peppermint flavor

Did Luke buy new toothpaste for me as a surprise?

This is a bad surprise

What the HECK?

Get it OUT OF MY MOUTH!

WHAT IN THE NAME OF LIFE is this STUFF??

WATER WATER WATER

DON'T SWALLOW

WHAT JUST HAPPENED??

DID I SWALLOW ANY OF IT?

IS MY THROAT GOING TO BE ON FIRE?

WHEN IS THIS GOING AWAY?

This isn't so bad now

My mouth sure does smell fresh

Whatever you do, don't do it. Just don't.

Random Thought:

Laughter is a great way to start your day.

63
MEET ME DISCOVERING ACUPUNCTURE

A year into treatment and I'm now reaching out to find more solutions. Top of the lists are Restorative Yoga and Acupuncture. A friend recommended a healing yoga salon and I contacted them by email to inquire if I might have a consultation before attending a first session. "You see," I wrote, "I have pelvic pain" and explained the symptoms, treatments, areas affected, and so forth. I thought this was best so they would have an idea of who I am and select poses to discuss. Promptly I received an email saying I was being referred over to the partner, but due to the fact that she was busy and worked full time, it might be a while before she would be able to respond. The tone was a little off and appeared like I was a problem already and we hadn't even met!

That evening I dove into research on restorative yoga on my laptop. I found articles, poses, breathing techniques and more. When yoga photos targeted problem muscles for me, I photographed them using my phone. My intent was to create a little guide I could refer to while I waited for this busy person to contact me back. The internet is a beautiful thing to help one bypass the annoyances of life and guide you to purposeful solutions.

I was now dragging one foot, I walked with caution, and coworkers were more than noticing the change in my stride and countenance. I was in pain. Little did I know that the poses I selected as restorative… really weren't. Alas, I did more damage to my IT band on my left leg than ever before. In fact, I could not move from bed one evening, nor could I move in bed either. What an agonizing day and night.

Not all things you research will work for you. Sigh.

In late January of 2017, I made an appointment with a new massage therapist for myofascial leg and hip treatments and to my surprise noticed she was also a certified acupuncturist. Three weeks later as I entered the massage room to undress and speak confidentially with her, I broke down sobbing. It had been a horrible day; my pain was high, my tolerance level was zero, and my faith in overcoming any semblance of life was vaporizing. "Do you do work in the pelvic area?" I inquired. Truthfully, I begged. Melody told me of research and success stories and, yes, she would like to help me. Thus started a new dimension to my treatment care.

I apologized for having to expose my full body to her. I was no longer modest but felt badly for her to work on body parts usually covered by underwear. Her calming nature quickly disseminated my anxiety and we got started. That evening after my first acupuncture session, my lower abdomen begun to loosen. This was the first time since May 2016 that I sensed hunger and I knew acupuncture was going to now be another key to the puzzle. It became apparent that if there was to be more success, acupuncture needed to be done twice a week for three months. Now with acupuncture and pelvic floor therapy combined to loosen and lengthen tight glutes, iliopsoas muscles, and a host of other muscles running from my diaphragm to my knees, I felt cautiously optimistic.

My brother was astounded when he discovered I utilized acupuncture and he had many questions. Do you get bloody? How long are the needles and how far do they go into the skin? Where do they put them? Is she Asian? What does it do? How long have you been going?

I have noticed a few things concerning acupuncture and that is the results come several hours afterwards and the releasing effects will be noticeable for a few days. If I go more than one week without acupuncture, the results fade. I would like to taper off as it is customary, but my body is not ready. I do not know the name of the points my acupuncturist uses but I trust her. Points near the ankle, inner thigh, a horseshoe shape from the outer thigh near the knee up and around my bottom and over and then down the other outer thigh. She also uses five points on the thumb and on the palm beneath the ring finger. We also use horizontal points which run across the bikini line in the pelvic area. She has placed needles near the nose for the release of body heat and at the top of the head for tension. Acupuncture is not covered by insurance but both Luke and I have agreed that because it works in releasing muscles and calming the nervous system, it's best I continue to add it into my treatment care. Melody has been a godsend. Her kindness and helping hands are genuine lifelines to me.

Random Thought:

Why do people complain about temporary inconveniences so much on social media?

64
MEET ME AND MY COPING SKILLS

Music is soothing and distracting. Listen to the words.

Heating pad. Buy an adaptor and keep one in your car, too.

Dragon ointment takes my mind off the abdomen and thighs.

Mugs with positive messages on them are great reminders.

Make a list of things to do and do one thing; mark it off to feel accomplished.

Get out of the house, scoot down on the porch chair, relax and prop up your legs. Feel the heat of the sun.

Do a kind deed for another.

Massage therapy and acupuncture work.

Light a candle and know you are worthy of petitioning God for healing.

Chiropractic visits may align the hips.

PT exercises at home are important.

Hot showers; take as many as needed.

Hammock time is divine.

Wine in between doses of medicine PRN. Wine relaxes the core.

Stroll outdoors as far as you can. Stroll indoors in the mall on bad weather days.

Keep a heating pad at work and cover it with a hoodie for privacy.

Practice RDS (Relax your body from the top of your head down to your toes. Drop your Pelvic Floor. Smile.)

Lean on a counter when your abdomen is tight and will not release.

Do not bleed your pain stories onto others.

Journal your thoughts.

Do not run out of medication; plan ahead.

Take day trips as tolerated.

Look for beauty and joyful things. They are still there.

Send cards to others.

Have a mantra to repeat to yourself on bad days.

Do not expect people to pick up your clues that you do not feel well.

You do not have Ultimate knowledge of how this is going to play out. Try not to fear the future.

Keep a diary of good things that happened as a result of your initiative. Look back later and realize you had a real purpose.

Distance yourself on bad days but don't isolate from others to an excess. You will miss blessings if you are alone too much.

A child's rubber, pointy ball makes a good massage tool on weary and tight muscles.

Watch National Geographic on television. It will expand your world.

Take special interest, close-up photos of items in your home. Find beauty in the most unexpected places. Make a scrapbook of these hidden gems.

Buy a heavy pillow and weigh yourself down with it. Press into your core. With butterfly thigh stretches, place the heavy pillow inside to hold the legs open without causing pressure.

Take your lunch and eat it outdoors.

Learn a new skill.

Wear a robe that is double-layered to keep the chills away.

Only do what you can do. Let things go. Ask for help. Resist the need to be independent.

Unfollow individuals on Facebook, as needed. Most people look happier with a delightfully fuller life than yours, or so it would appear, when they post.

Do not feel the need to explain yourself. If you cannot attend an event and others want to know why, simply reply, "Thank you for caring for me."

Art therapy.

Break a task into divisions you can accomplish.

Buy protein powder and keep yogurt in the refrigerator. On days you do not have an appetite, a smoothie will offer nutrition.

Expect to lose some weight but don't get too alarmed. You are still healthy; it's the muscle war that is the problem.

Shop in smaller increments of time. Utilize the internet.

Simplify the holidays.

Burn candles and use a warmer. The occasional new aromas will delight your senses.

Use spell check before sending an email or text. Your brain is fighting as hard as your body. Spelling and grammar mistakes will be both comical and more prevalent.

Confide in a priest, pastor, or spiritual mentor.

Float in water.

Open Spaces: visualize your pelvic area opening. Sit on a toilet while putting your shoes, socks, or panties and tights on. Your bottom will love the open feeling. Visualize open spaces that have brought you delight: spring time in an open field, an open airy lakeside picnic, the vastness and openness of a ski resort atop a mountain, the solitude and openness while walking and laying on a beach. Remember how your body responds as you drive out of a large city, leaving the metal, concrete, tons of asphalt behind you and begin to encounter less traffic. You exhale. Your eyes adjust to the openness of the surrounding of the countryside: open fields, vast forests, endless plains. Utilize visual 3D virtual reality headsets to reduce pain. CDs are available which take you on a visual path of healing and relaxation.

65
MEET ME WITH LAUGHTER

I had not seen a precious friend named Valerie in a long time. Using an old cell phone number, I texted:

"Hello, I'll be up there on Monday and would you be available to get together then?"

She didn't respond right away. She had lost my number through the years and my name and number registered as an unknown caller on her cell phone screen. I then began to worry. "OH NO, I have waited too long! She has a new number. Or she has moved out of state. Will I ever see my friend again? Oh, why oh, why did I wait so long?"

Thankfully, Valerie wrote back and we made quick arrangements and both excitedly looked forward to reconnecting. What a joy! After a medical appointment along with physical therapy, we met nearby for lunch. She asked why I was coming all this distance for physical therapy. There was no short answer to that question! I told her the basic truth. She empathized and I knew she shared my burden. But lunch was not centered on me. We had a good time catching up, relating with similar family scenarios, and laughing together but eating little because we spent most of our time talking and listening. When it was time to depart, we asked the busboy to take our picture. He was more than willing to accommodate our wishes but stated emphatically he was a horrible photographer. With a smartphone how can this be? Certainly, he was wrong. Within minutes of our picture being taken, we looked at the photo and agreed. It was the worst photo either of us could have taken, and not social media worthy!

But after returning home and reflecting upon our special grownup play date with one another, I looked intently at the photo. We both had our eyes closed due to laughter. We were two friends, connected by love and history, captured in the worst possible second for a Polaroid moment but it was the best frozen memory in time I could have asked for. We were laughing and smiling, gazing at one another, and sharing the best gift we had to offer – priceless appreciation and heartfelt devotion. As it was, it turned out to be one of my favorite photos.

Random Thought:

The best things in life are warm hugs, meaningful relationships, deep faith, and genuine smiles.

66
MEET ME AT THE HOT TUB

Mentally I wrote on my meager-sized bucket list: Spend the night by myself in a hotel. Just Me, Myself, and I. My family members and most of my friends and work associates had done this and thought nothing of it. However, I had no reason, nor desire to spend money on myself in this fashion before. It seemed a little exorbitant, selfish, and a tad bit anti-social to express my desire to go off alone and hibernate for 24 hours, much less carry through with the plans.

Several months prior, I had scheduled two medical appointments in the city and at the time thought it was going to be a perfect time to take advantage of a getaway with my husband, find out some good news from the professionals, and enjoy the luxury of a nice hotel with its number one amenity: a hot tub.

However, a week prior to the appointments and in my desire to improve my flexibility and strength I overdid it. Not intentionally but, ultimately, I didn't know what the heck I was doing. Believe me, I tried to understand what my body needed and I explored many yoga poses I believed my body could do at an adaptive level. I googled, studied photos with precise movements and set out to be restored through yoga. This was the key!

In an earlier time, I had taken yoga, Pilates, cardio workouts, cycling, step classes, played tennis (badly, but I played), walked, swam, jogged and hiked, but my all-time favorite was aerobics to music. The rhythmic movements and music were a beautiful synchronization to keep muscles toned and to build strength. I will admit even back then, yoga was foreign to my body. My strained hips would not open and stretch like other participants. Now I understand why. I must have been born with hip dysplasia but merely didn't know it.

Back to restorative yoga. With dedication, I worked with finding poses my body could do and selected eight to ten. I began to feel tighter. This seemed reasonable since my body had been "at rest" for a year with no exercise; this was to be expected. I should expect a little rebellion. The next evening after work, I went through the restorative yoga patterns again. Evening after evening I practiced until I began limping, then I couldn't stand on my left leg unassisted. A few days later I could hardly maneuver myself in and out of the front seat of my car. "What is happening?" I cried out inwardly. "The more I try, the more my body fails me."

In desperation, I YouTubed (I believe this is a verb now!) several massage techniques designed to release the iliopsoas muscles and tight IT Band and connective tissues running down my left leg from my hip to the knee. I showed Luke and asked him to watch the video and then to work on me. He knows anatomy more than I as he took it in college and has been an athlete for years. Plus, I knew he wouldn't hurt me.

I was back to square one after our five-minute session and this time I could not move. I was in excruciating pain. Doubling up on muscle relaxers, a bit of wine, a couple of pain pills from a family member, two heating pads and remaining in bed finally released those muscles many hours later. I couldn't go to the bathroom because I couldn't bend my leg. Solution: I would choose not to drink anything so I wouldn't need to get out of bed. I slept with the offending leg dangling off the side of the bed, supported by pillows and tied to the opposite thigh by a soft bathrobe sash to keep it from slipping. Lord have mercy, what a night.

After this pandemonium in my body, I didn't know if I could make it to my hotel room. I was disappointed and felt exhausted in knowing how to make any manner of plans again. Ever. No Plans Amy. NPA. But I began to feel stronger and Luke and I agreed a hotel stay in a luxury suite with a Jacuzzi would do me good. The joy in knowing I could make a few plans and carry them out was reviving! CHEERS – can you hear them?

At the hot tub, ten minutes upon arrival, I had eased myself into the hot bubbly waters and was literally soaking it all in. This is it. I'm so thankful. There was a sign on the adjacent wall which clarified the optimal time spent in a hot tub was 15 minutes. Forget that, baby. This girl is not getting out until she is good and ready. After 20 minutes of pure relaxation, a lady joined me. I noticed her out of the corner of my eye when she hopped over and into the hot tub. I didn't pay attention to the details as I was in my own world.

We both concurred this hotel was exceptional in décor and amenities, and then casually mentioned what had brought each other here. I soon realized I was in the pool with a celebrity of the worst nightmare in Oklahoma history. The domestic terrorist truck bombing attack at the Alfred P. Murrah Federal Building on April 19, 1995 changed the course of history. I had read her story and the memories came flooding back as she simply said that she was the one who had been trapped in the Social Security Office on the first floor and her leg was amputated to save her life. What she didn't say in the hot tub was she had also lost her mother, her three-year old child and infant. Instead she introduced me to her miracle child, her son who had been born one year later. Life has been hard since then. She would have loved to have had a life filled with a career and, more, to be pain and flashback free, but instead had lived these twenty plus years on disability and with a family member. Doing her best despite the horrific details that rained on her 22 years ago are now the constants in her life. She wasn't defined by her circumstances; she didn't introduce herself by saying, "I'm the woman who had my leg cut off with an Exacto knife in the basement of the Murrah building" but instead mildly spoke of an upcoming interview that had brought her to this hotel.

I'm so sorry for your loss. Why do I carry grief in my heart for the body I now have when your life was literally changed forever? Yet, you graciously carry on, my new friend.

I saw her at breakfast the next morning and told her how much she had inspired me. We held hands and looked deep into each other's eyes and connected. With God's Heart, I love you too, Daina Bradley.

Random Thought:

Be kind and accepting for all acts of kindnesses shown to you during this time of healing. It's not the gift that is given; it's the thought and reminder you are deeply loved. People care for you. They may not know what to say or what to offer, but their intent is to relieve a bit of pain. What would you give to someone in your shoes?

67
MEET ME AS A SNOWFLAKE

A young adult friend who is surprisingly inquisitive and creative in many aspects of her life loves to capture the beauty of individual snowflakes as they fall. Elena is an accomplished photographer, although photography is but one of many hobbies. She could turn it into a profitable business had she not chosen the path of education first and foremost. Why she captures the beauty of snowflakes is of grand mystery. She absolutely hates to be cold and wears boots, leggings and sweatshirts even in summer. However, Elena will muster the fortitude to withstand the cold for long periods of time in the anticipation of capturing at most a few fallen ornaments from God. "It is the craziest thing to see all the intricate designs and detail put into individual snowflakes. How much more designed and thought out we must be." This life-loving friend shares her glimpses of God's love to us through social media.

I returned to the Botanical Gardens this morning and hanging from the highest rafters were colossal, ornamental snowflakes. Man made of course, but it brought back her words into focus. The phrases "I am loved" and "intricately created" resounded in my mind several times that morning. I needed reassurance. Working to stretch and retrain my body to work in unity and to harmonize within itself is my #1 goal. I do not feel intricately made when pain hits hard. I do not feel loved when I'm not sure my prayers for healing will be answered. I KNOW He can but will he choose to or not?

I am a Snowflake

Am I on a solitary path that is unique for me?

Will I become more of my true self during this process?

Am I becoming more loving and intuitive with others?

Do I see beauty in new and divine ways?

Can I find peace, fulfillment and joy in this journey?

Am I able to accept this as a journey of one?

68
MEET ME AND THE RUNNERS

A s I look out the sweeping windows facing the streets of downtown, I see a couple of guys run by and think, "Wow, they must be exceptionally late for work if they are running that fast." A few more minutes pass and here comes another man in black pants and a red polo shirt. This is intriguing. "Where are these guys going and why are they so dressed up? Who runs in black slacks and red polo shirts? Oh, I hope an emergency of some kind isn't down the street!" Time passes as I sip my coffee and unexpectedly here comes another red polo shirted guy running by! "Well, this is too coincidental. Is this a running club that requires their members to in business/casual attire?" I've got to find out.

Upon inquiring, I discover these young men are not in a running club and not on an emergency drill of any kind. Surprisingly, they are employees of the hotel and work in the valet parking department. I am super impressed with the enthusiasm for their job. "Who knew that parking cars could have such an impact?"

I've never enjoyed running. My heart raced; I gasped for air. When I ran, I missed the details of the path. I was too focused on my pace, breathing correctly, and trying to make it to the next mark. I much preferred power walking. But although I was not a runner, I did run. I ran from one activity to another. My calendar was full. Every hour was given to some activity, chore, person, event, and/or contribution of one kind or another. I was accountable and responsible and enjoyed making my moments and days count for something good. I had the energy to do it and felt compelled to make life better for the people around me. I volunteered, cheered them on, worked, cleaned, and was the traditional power woman that many are today: wife, mom, nurse, housecleaner, launderer, taxi, party planner, boo-boo comforter, cheerleader, decorator of all things, advocate, educator, religious instructor, date night organizer and still found time for creating memories for loved ones, indoors and out. I loved being involved and I loved being alive. I forfeited television for spending time with my children and husband instead.

I did not anticipate stopping. Of course, I knew my life would change as my children grew up and moved away but then I would begin the cycle again with grandchildren. I had no final chapter written in my mind. I was the energizer bunny who planned to keep going.

I don't run anymore from activity to activity but I do have a new sense of acceptance of events and activities I can participate in. I savor them. I appreciate time spent in memorable and meaningful activities and discussions with friends and family. I rely on social media to engage with people when I can't be there in person. I have slowed down and now make my fewer activities I can do just as meaningful. I am learning to be flexible and spontaneous, and to appreciate events that come as bursts of joy and love. This is my new strategy.

This new pathway is not for runners; it is for walkers. I am willing to walk and believe and to celebrate what is waiting at the bend of the road.

69
MEET ME UNCLOTHED

These past fourteen months have been the most "open" time of my entire life. I have not lain on this many examining tables, undressed, nor had professionals touch this, that and the other as much as during this time period. I've never discussed hygiene, constipation, and specific lady parts and what they look and feel like with anyone. ANYONE. Until now. My world has changed and I am both drowning and soaking in it – depends on the day.

I'm trying to love my body in a new way. I'm laying here typing this chapter naked. Yes, NAKED.

I'm exploring this concept. My appearance is not up for inspection as I know what I look like and don't feel badly it. Nakedness today is not in reference to sexiness, either. It's more in respect to the lack of restraint, I suppose. My mission is to sink deeply into myself and to relax my mind, body, and spirit and to see where this takes me. Will my pelvic muscles ever relax? I am told I have eight muscle groups incorporated in this affliction that operates as a domino effect, each influencing the other.

Release. Relax. Just Be.

It's essential I love myself. I've never been so vulnerable in my entire life.

70

MEET ME AND MY FRIEND ANGELA

T his past year, I received weekly phone calls from a new friend. I say this with a smile and hint of sarcasm as it is not a "real person" who is calling me, but an electronic answering machine. Angela is enthusiastic! Although I have memorized the script, I listen all the way through, just in case she has new information to share with me.

"Hello, this is the Pelvic Pain Clinic located at 2110 N.W. Broadway, Suite G calling to remind (pause) Amy of a scheduled appointment on Tuesday, May 23rd at 3 pm. It is VERY important for you to contact us at 504 – 753 – 8545 if you are unable to keep this scheduled appointment. Failure to show may result in a no-show fee. Please bring a photo ID, your current insurance card, list of medications, and any payment currently due. We look forward to seeing you. Thank you for choosing Pelvic Pain Clinic."

I have become accustomed to receiving this voice message and am not annoyed by them. Each is reassuring to me. I have a place to go and they want me there. Simple as that. I believe it's okay to have a "friend" who calls weekly to offer friendly reminders; in fact, I have given her a name. Her name is Angela, which means messenger. It's all in our perspective.

71
MEET ME ON A BAD DAY

There have been too many bad days and I don't want to remember them, in their intense description, in their deviousness of stealing my joy, and in their fierce and unrelenting agony they have caused. My optimistic spirit and my fun-filled focus on life are nonexistent on bad days. But I will remember them because they are now a part of me, and I pledge to use my experiences to help another. I promise not to forget; there are people who need a kindred spirit on their bad day.

I will not forget.

On bad days, people are louder.

On bad days, cabinet door slams are more offensive.

On bad days, I drop more things.

On bad days, I groan when I stand up.

On bad days, I move more slowly.

On bad days, I need more rest.

On bad days, food is not appealing.

On bad days, I feel left out.

On bad days, my face looks old.

On bad days, I take more showers.

On bad days, I can't see tomorrow.

On bad days, I do the best I can.

Random thought:

Thank you, dear family, for giving me privacy and respecting my need for space.

72
MEET ME AND THE BIG BLOWOUT

*W*arning: This is ugly

Once upon a time, my husband planned an escape for me during this time of distress. He texted Christine with reference to a possible mini-vacation during Spring Break. YES, of course! She was all in! The two communicated back and forth during the afternoon and put preliminary details together.

The trip was to be multi-functional. She and Eduardo had purchased their first home together in late 2016. Luke and I had enjoyed the photos but were longing to visit and see the home in person. Traveling had been out of the question thus far. Indeed, Luke and I had planned to travel to Destin mid-summer and in his line of thinking, this would be a trial to see how my body responded to driving, catching a flight, and enjoying a few days out of town.

"Would it be possible to also go to the beach?" Luke and Christine both wondered. Well, of course, mom LOVES the beach and it's within an hour's drive.

Perfect. Except it wasn't.

Oh my, it would be interesting to see a full video replay of the following episode as it later unfolded in our living room.

"Amy, when you have time, I want to talk to you about something."

"I'll be done in 15 or 20 minutes. I'm balancing the checkbook."

Lying on the couch later while my husband was in his recliner, casually watching a basketball game on TV, I asked, "What did you want to talk about?"

From there on he began to deliberately outline details of a possible mini-vacation in four weeks. As he lovingly portrayed the thoughtfulness of each decision he and our daughter had considered, the panic rose, inch by inch in my now trembling body. I covered up with a blanket and focused on calming techniques, trying to maintain my focus that they were doing this for me and to get a grip. Relax. "There was no way," I thought. As the details continued to emerge, the more I felt backed into a corner like a scared cat with no escape route. Finally (or so it felt) there was silence. My turn.

"Christine and Eduardo go out to eat every single night! That means driving to a location 30 minutes away, waiting in crowded restaurants for a table, sitting for over an hour, driving back to their home and that's just for one crazy meal! And you two want to extend this mini-vacation now to FOUR DAYS? I have been there with her. You get stuck in traffic! It's normal for them but it will KILL ME to sit that long in a car! And you guys can TOTALLY FORGET about driving to the beach!! I have driven it and the drive is not 45 minutes. Traffic backs up the closer you get to the island!! Just getting to her house from the stinking airport is going to set my body off! I CAN'T DO IT!!" I screamed.

I didn't even mention the fact that leaving after work on a Friday, driving 85 miles to an airport, catching a flight which I had NO IDEA how my body would react to in a vibrating seat that bounced along with turbulence, arriving to our destination late at night, more driving, and then finally getting to their house at almost midnight was beyond INSANE. And that was at the beginning of this so-called vacation!

They were proud of their plan. I was smoldering.

HIM: "You aren't even listening. This is only an option."

ME: "No it's not. You guys spent all afternoon planning it. Every time I went near the recliner you were texting each other."

HIM: "YOU ARE SO NEGATIVE!"

ME: "YOU HAVE NO IDEA WHAT IT'S LIKE TO BE ME! TAKE SOMEONE ELSE ON THE VACATION! I CAN'T GO!"

SLAM DOORS

HIM: "DON'T YOU EVER SLAM A DOOR IN MY FACE AGAIN!"

ME: "GET OUT GET OUT GET OUT"

Shower time with lots of sobbing. How in the world could my family possibly believe I could handle this? I'm invisible to them. Luke plainly wants a vacation. This was a nice day, too. It's ruined now. How dare they go and plan a vacation under the pretense of it's "for me" when they don't even know me. They know the old me. They have NO IDEA who the new me is. I don't even know who I am anymore

Later: I'm reading and lying on a heating pad. Alone. Luke comes in and sits on the floor. We attempt to communicate our intentions but it rates a D+ on the conversational/truly listening scale. He walks away.

"I think I will go live by myself."

"No, you won't," he says.

"You have no idea, buddy, how wrong you might be," I say to myself.

Time lapse 48 hours later and we are finally able to discuss this situation in an adult manner. He writes me a letter and I write back. Pain has stolen any resemblance of emotional cushion and I was more than ever wiped out. Up until this journey of pain and healing, I understood I was alone but I thought I at least had depth of understanding from those closest to me. When it was stripped away, true ugly came pouring out. It was one of the most frightful evenings in my life to feel totally alone.

A woman I met later confided to me she had Multiple Sclerosis and her husband doesn't get it all the time. We cannot expect anyone, including our spouses, to completely understand our every thought and action. I was expecting too much from my husband and the primal instinct of fear and anger came bursting out without any holds or constraints. For better or for worse. Our wedding vows were promised one to another 35 years ago and we meant them.

But.

Marriage is hard sometimes.

Random Thought:

I will listen to "Even If" by Mercy Me again tonight. This song is my prayer for healing and peace; when I don't see the way, I will still take a stand.

73
MEET ME AND MY HAIR

O n March 2011, my husband and I were in the Atlanta, Georgia airport. We had arrived from 900 miles away and were there for a layover to another destination. As we hurried through the terminal I observed a robed priest and various individuals as they walked briskly up to him, lowered their eyes, and then received a marking on his/her forehead. Short prayers were quietly observed from the hundreds of passersby, including me. Obviously, something was going on.

I asked myself, "Were we under high terrorist alert and was I the only one who didn't know? Why would random individuals beseech an unknown robed priest and voluntarily request that gray colored copier toner stuff be smeared on their foreheads?"

I was at a loss. Luke looked at me like I was crazy, and admonished, "Don't you know - it's Ash Wednesday. I believe in this case they are asking the priest for prayers of protection as well as observing the beginning of Lent."

Oh, now that makes sense. Maybe I could ask for prayers of protection, too. I had at no time ever celebrated or even understood the complexities of Lent. I did have limited knowledge that a person would give up something in exchange for concentrating on the real meaning of Easter. Lent lasts close to 45 days and the things my friends and others had given up previously sounded a bit hokey to me. M&Ms were an all-time favorite during my teenage years.

I wondered even then, "Do you seriously think God cares if you eat M&Ms?"

Fast Forward to April 2016. The last time my hair had been colored with shades of golden strands and soft brown undertones, then conditioned and stylishly trimmed was in January. I love having my hair done. I adore my stylist and her salon with its adjoining boutique. The relaxing atmosphere is a true component to the spa ambience. To then sit under heat is pure bliss all in its own. After three hours of total relaxation and not worrying one ounce of what may be transpiring in the outside world is true pleasure.

But now sitting is difficult. I must change positions every twenty minutes and I alternate between lying, reclining, standing, stretching, and others. I cannot fathom being in one place for a full three hours. I'm uncommonly private now, and conversations are short. I cannot tolerate listening to others for long, and by long, I mean more than ten minutes. Without thinking any further, I dismissed making hair appointments and preceded to trim my bangs and then the full length of hair when it became necessary.

A few more months went by and now my roots were up front and center. There was no disguising the fact my hairstyle was evolving into a new one. It wasn't intentional; it was out of necessity. One morning while looking at myself in the mirror, it occurred I am observing the sacred practice of relinquishing a tangible object of life for Lent. I have chosen to give up my hair. My hair is there but it's not gone this long without expertise and care. Probably ever, I realize. As I look in the mirror each day, I see the new me gazing back. The new me who is fighting with all she possesses to maintain her sanity in this new world of chronic pain. This new world of uncertainty.

I have given up my hair, which is a tangible reminder these roots are the time rings of the pain and stress I have endured. These are my battle scars and these are my prayers. I have suffered but I have endured. And I will continue to endure with God's help; I am an overcomer in this private and solitary place of time and identity I did not choose for myself. I see myself as changing and my longer hair, which now has strands of gray wisps, are cries to God from my soul to please see me and heal me. I am fasting. This is my Lent. This is not some kind of frivolous and childish game of relinquishing M&Ms for 45 days. This is my life we are talking about.

I believe I am going to be healed. I repeat the words "This is not forever" over and over in my mind and to my aching body. It's a prayer and a personal commitment that I will hold fast. I will continue to believe.

I am unsure of what I will do with my hair; my crown. I may choose to wear it long the rest of my life to ensure I don't forget. I have withstood and evolved. My hair is my private memorial of pain, prayers, and thanksgiving for provision. One night I dreamed my hair was waist long and curled at the ends. I didn't notice the color and, if I did, I couldn't recall it upon waking. I don't know if I was healed or not. But I looked happy.

Random Thought:

Trust your instincts.

74
MEET ME AFTER PT

I love my PT gals. What must they be thinking after I leave? Do I make an impression of any kind? My appointment is scheduled for the last one of the day and no doubt they are ready to return to their families. There must be days each wishes she could leave the parking lot a bit earlier. Traffic is the beast! But do they think of me after I leave?

I would like for them to see me as the girl who tries so hard.

The mom who cares for her family more than life itself.

The employee who won't leave work early in exchange for an earlier appointment.

The wife and husband team who drive up together even when other husbands often drift away.

Does Olivia wonder what crazy thing I am going to try next?

Do they believe I am overreacting or underreacting?

I love listening to them talk about their own lives. Do they enjoy the stories I tell?

Do they in hushed tones discuss when I leave that I'm not as far along as I should be?

Does Dr. Hannah worry I may give up?

Are they sorry my pace of improvement is slow?

Are Dr. Hannah and Olivia proud of me?

Will we be friends when this is over?

Will it ever be over?

This is my solitary journey, but I feel less alone when I am with them. It's the most optimistic hour of my week. They are my lights but do they know how brightly they shine for me?

Random Thought:

"The prevalence of nonrelaxing pelvic floor disorders is unknown. The underlying mechanism for this phenomenon is poorly understood." (Recognition and Management of Nonrelaxing Pelvic Floor Dysfunction by Stephanie S. Faubion, Lynne T. Shuster, and Adil E. Bharucha. www. ncbi.nlm.nih.gov.) Thank you for laying it out on the line with the truth.

75

MEET ME AND MY DAD

On April 13, 2017, I posted on Facebook: "I'd like to tell you about my dad. He is now giving lectures once a week to medical students on the topics of ministry through health, various religious practices and how they influence a person's hospital stay, and practical knowledge on how to utilize chaplains. He is 86 years old. Proud of you dad." Then I uploaded a joyful photo of him and mom.

Forty-seven friends "liked" this post, eleven positive comments were written, and one person shared the post on their own timeline. It was amazing to see the number of people who were touched by this disclosure. I meant to forward the positive information to him; he deserved to read the overwhelming responses he had received on behalf of my sharing his story. But I didn't.

Then dad did another remarkable thing. He joined Facebook himself! We became "friends" and on May 23rd I woke up to a text message from him saying he had discovered the post and was deeply touched. He had decided it was his obligation to keep moving and doing and living and giving to others.

If dad searched into the depths of my timeline, he would have seen quite a gap in time. I had become frustrated by the prognosis for improvement after the discovery of hip dysplasia and the affirmation I might not be able to completely heal. I was focused on my disastrous year and I, in a temporarily fit of grief and anger one evening, began reevaluating the past. As I scrolled through my timeline, I deleted one post after another. Delete. Delete. Delete. I wanted this year covered up, gone, dead and buried. I wanted no record of it.

My posts were without a doubt 100 percent positive. I was, and will continue to be, an encourager. I try to see the good and happy side of life. On my timeline you won't find mention of city turmoil, localized crime, or statewide obstruction of any kind. This was the year for politics if there ever was one! I don't gripe and complain on Facebook. I don't disclose too much and you will have to look long and hard to find posts I wish I had not written. There was no reason to dispose of the media traces of my life. What kept me from wiping out the entire year were photos of my grandchildren I had posted. They are the only tangible evidence I even existed on Facebook during the past 12 months.

Did the delete fit satisfy me? No. Did that act of self-sabotage take away any negative emotions I still carried in my heart? No. Do I even know why I attempted to wipe out the footprints of my life? Not really.

Sometimes no explanation comes to mind.

But I'm still here, and my goal is to "keep moving and doing and living and giving to others." Just like dad.

Random Thought:

"You have been assigned this mountain to show others it can be moved." - UNKNOWN

76
MEET ME WITH THE MEDS

W hat has saved my life this year is a muscle relaxant. However, it has come with huge pitfalls – namely, it knocked me out. This is a good thing if it is bedtime but in my situation I needed it while working as a resource specialist. This was a problem. The capsule was time-released and was to be taken with water every five hours. Here was my scenario. Wake up: take a capsule and hopefully at the one-hour mark when I would dip into my first zombie status as it activated, I had completed morning announcements by intercom and instruction time with first hour had concluded. As students implemented the lesson in the computer lab, I would make my way to a chair to regain momentum. Dropping out was not an option; I had to keep functioning. By 11 am my body was screaming for another dose but it was not yet time. I must endure one more hour. Noon: take another capsule but I would feel no release from pain until it activated 60 minutes later. Forget about eating lunch. At 1 pm I would begin to feel a bit better and could make it through the end of the school day. By the time I arrived home, the pain was again climbing higher so I would either drink a glass of wine, take a Valium Suppository to relax internal muscles, or both. Laying in the backroom on a heating pad I would slip into a coma. Living was exhausting. Luke prepared most of his evening meals as I often slept until 7 pm. The rest of our evening would be spent relaxing or doing physical therapy. My final capsule at bedtime would send me into a good night's rest.

Over and over. The nightmare with no ending.

In early spring after returning from a "sit in my car during a lunch date with myself," I was zoned out. The officer on duty looked directly into my eyes and asked how I was doing. It was at that point I realized how close I was to becoming seen as an impaired employee. Prescription meds, no less, but not fit to work here. I'm so thankful it did not come to a site investigation. How humiliating that would have been to be whisked off to take a drug test, and it would have severed my dream of finishing strong.

Then I discovered in late spring of 2017 this muscle relaxant, which also came in tablet form, could be broken in half and taken every two hours. The tablet required food so I was now required to eat six times a day. Since I had lost 12% of my body weight, this seemed like a good solution. This regime of six half tablets instead of three capsules lessened the steep dip of its effects and kept the pain at a more tolerable level.

As my muscles subdued, and my ability to walk further increased, I grew more hopeful in early summer of 2017. The peripheral neuropathy, however, was still the plague and I set out to find more information. Research led me to the conclusion I needed an antidepressant. I discovered with chronic pain, endorphins are used up in the same pathway as pain signals and antidepressants can help. This antidepressant also offered a decrease in nerve firing sensations; the feeling of ants crawling on my feet, bee stings throughout my legs, and vise grip holds from the groin to my calf muscles were wearing me out. Another medication I asked for was Lidocaine ointment, prescription strength. I began to tally my good days with how many applications of lidocaine were needed per day. A one application day was a day to celebrate!

Eight years ago, I remember Dr. A suggested I take an antidepressant and discontinue the use of HRT. Many of my menopausal symptoms might be alleviated, he stated. At that moment, I revealed, "Why would I do that? I'm the sanest person in my family!" Boy oh boy, if he could see me now. What a lively discussion we would have!

Random Thought:

Garth Brooks came to town and he was within a reasonable driving distance. Not once, twice, three, but four times Garth crashed downtown Oklahoma City in a mighty way and sent the state reeling in good vibes and with state pride during his four impressive concerts. After all, Garth was a product of Oklahoma State University, a bona fide member of the Sooner State, and he was a beloved musical endorsement that great things do come from Oklahoma.

I had settled the issue when the tickets went on sale for the big events. "Amy," I said, "You can just as easily listen to his songs at home, forgo the voucher price, not be jostled by loud and adrenalized ticket stub holders, unnecessarily walk or stand for hours, nor sit in uncomfortable stadium seating, and by no means sit in a car for 200 miles when the day is over."

"Good idea," I said to myself. However...

My sound decision-making skills started slipping and sliding into the murky green waters of the envy pool. I'm now familiar with the algae filled pool which is surrounded by huge trees, covered over in creeping, life-sucking green moss which hangs, drips, and overtakes life in its path. Green is a bad place.

"Help!" I called. "I'm going under and I need a lifeline to get me out!"

The best way to climb out of the pool of envy is to remind yourself that no one has it all, discern that life is not a competition, and to focus on gratitude instead.

77
MEET ME WITH A GREETING CARD

In our world of education, gaining cheers and high fives from ALL students is an impossibility. However, Gala certainly gains respect by the majority. She is devoted, specific in goals, inspiring, and is a true leader by creating a climate in which students can count on achieving successful outcomes. She did all this, daily, hour after hour, while being in pain. She often limped, slumped, and moved at a slower pace to restore her aching muscles which created much havoc from a long, accepted disease. Gala was my inspiration to keep going and not let it catch up with you. One day, I decided to send her a notecard. I wrote inside:

"I wanted to tell you what a blessing you have been to me, as I see you face life's physical struggles with courage! Your medical tools of massage, positivity on Facebook, relying on God – all with a smile on your face 99% of the time is sometimes the only thing that gets me through one moment to another. I, too suffer from chronic pain, which I woke up to on February 7th. God has a plan and is using this physical nightmare to place me in a position of total dependency on Him. I was told I will see relief in six to twelve months for this rare muscular, skeletal, and nerve issue after it was diagnosed in June, but it will/or may be a part of my new normal the rest of my life. Thank you for lighting the way in my new journey as I have had to redefine what a 'good day' looks like. Hugs, My Friend."

78
MEET ME AND THE CHAIR

I have decided to keep the reason for my retirement a secret. Well, not totally a secret as my family, ladies group, a few friends at work, and the Bon Temps know. In the school district where I work, Board notes are published once or twice a month, depending upon the number of meetings that were held. Following the minutes are the Human Resource listings of those who were hired, relocated, leaving, retiring, or were terminated. Once my name gets on this list, the word will be out. I believe it will be published in early April.

To my surprise, my job posted on the website in March before my name appeared in the Retiring column of the April Board notes. As word circulated, the first question I heard was: "You are retiring?" as if this must be a mistake, then followed by a series of comments and questions.

"You are too young!"

"What will you do?"

"You don't look old enough to retire!"

"Insurance. You know it's expensive. I had to find another job just to pay for mine."

"Who's going to replace you? It's never going to be the same."

"Are you sure you are retiring?"

As I nodded and smiled, I then waited to hear their advice because I knew it was coming.

"When I retired from civil service, I painted, organized, and volunteered. After nine months, I became bored and was asked to work as a tutor. I know you will want to find something like this."

"So, what are you going to do now?"

"Ah, you're a grandmother so you will enjoy those babies so much. You know you can come back with a part time job though, don't you?"

"Seriously, what are you going to do?"

Believe me, I have thought of these things, and more. I listened to their advice, their personal stories, and read their eyes and welcomed their hugs as they genuinely cared for me. Perspective. My coworkers wanted the best for me. Thank you, friends.

Why did I not share my true reasons for retirement? I could have easily replied: "I have an ailment. I now live in pain. This has been the most difficult year of my life. It took courage to get out of bed each morning. I can't keep up with this pace." For years I had laughingly told the head custodian who fussed at me for climbing upon a chair to hang decorations: "When I can't climb on a chair any longer, I will know it's time to retire."

Coworkers and friends, my legs and hips are no longer strong and steady. I can't climb in a chair with the assurance I have done my entire career. It's time to let go of the past and prepare for the future. It's been a process all year of leaving education and saying goodbye to my crazy, incredible, and stressful but abundantly rewarding career. But thank you for your love and care for me. It means the world.

Can I count the many changes I have had in life? Of course not. No one is ever stuck for long; change is always just beyond the corner.

79

MEET ME DECLARING I AM NOT A VACANCY

I received quite a shock when a teacher stepped into my office and incidentally stated "since you are retiring…" I was stunned. Three employees knew and he wasn't one of them. After stewing, I decided to announce my retirement on a closed Facebook group for my school. It's my party and I can do what I want to! I was amazed at the support that followed. The piece was a bit like an obituary you would write yourself but then had the pleasure of reading. I highly recommend it!

"Word will be spreading soon of a new opportunity next fall. To my astonishment, an unexpected detour has surfaced and I will be retiring a bit earlier than I had planned. I will be excited to hear how the resource center develops with new ideas and thoughtful preparations for our students and you in mind. This has been my home for 24 years. How interesting I have had quite unexpected bookends at the beginning and now at the end of my career. Before I signed a contract with HR years ago, I received this information: We have had a bit of misfortune and must now offer you the job at ¾ of the pay for two years. But at the beginning of the third year, your wages will be on track. Would you still like to accept the job? With providence I will complete this year with a final bookend called persistent pain. This detour is a bit hard to accept but aren't we all on our own personal journeys? We learn the hardest lessons with difficulty.

In between the bookends I have had so much joy. My best advice is to save your own sweet notes of appreciation, your best lessons, any advertising that made the newspaper, articles from the school news-letters, which highlight your accomplishments, and photos. One day you will each have enough material to fill a scrapbook with beautiful memories from a career few can relate to these days. My scrapbooks will be my anchors in the days ahead.

Transitions are a bit difficult; I hate long goodbyes and am horrified at the thought of crying in public places! I wanted to share this info as late as possible but word is getting out and I already know of two candidates for this upcoming position. Love and hugs to all!"

Reactions were quick and humbling; here is a sampling.

Congratulations on your retirement and the many things you have accomplished!

We admire and respect the things you have done for our school, the students, and the staff.

I will miss all your support and hearing your great ideas.

I have admired your creativity, compassion for others, and energy!

Thank you for being an anchor in the building and the calm when it was sometimes stormy. Thank you for being Johnny on the Spot with resources, ideas, suggestions, and a listening ear.

Thank you for being my friend.

Enjoy the next chapter of your book!

You allowed your students to grow academically and your inspiring and creative activities helped them to grow into young leaders.

Pelvic Pain Rehab Blog www.pelvicpainrehab.com/blog

I have admired your positive outlook and never-ending hard work.

Good luck, sweet friend, you have touched many lives. I wish you the best on your next journey in life.

The seeds you have planted in students who have passed through will continue to bloom their entire life.

You are such a tremendous inspiration and positive influence for many young lives. You are an irreplaceable legacy.

I have loved working with you so much.

You are an amazing, caring, and thoughtful person.

Your spirit will not be forgotten. I will miss you.

Thank you, dear friends. I am deeply humbled.

Random Thought:

Often, blessings cannot be received unless we go through the trial of waiting.

80
MEET ME AND THE LIFE LESSONS

What has this dysfunction taught me? Predominantly the saying, "You never know a man until you have walked in his shoes" has new meaning. Compassion works. Judgment doesn't.

I look beyond the actions of others and am more solution-minded instead.

I now better understand Claire, who has a cruel disease. When she was diagnosed at the age of thirteen, we had not even known of this disease much less understood its lifetime impact. If we had never heard of it, it couldn't be too bad, right? Wrong. As the years followed, through the highs and lows, with medication trial and error, multiple hospitalizations and surgeries, loss of school days and workdays, and pain filled nights to name a few, I assured my daughter I would go through this disease with her. She would not be alone. When she was on an elimination diet or liquid diet, I ate and drank what she did. When she physically could not attend events, I encouraged but did not insist. The many times she was on Prednisone for extended periods, I insisted she was beautiful. When she was raging inside, I let her be. I felt like I had been there for her and we had bonded through shared experiences.

Now I can relate on a new level of understanding. I know the fear that comes with chronic illness. I know the loneliness with perceptions of feeling forgotten. I know what it feels like to feel different and to be different. Fatigue is an enemy, which is a thief that can win, temporarily, and I understand this. Isolation is another prison. Please forgive me, sweet girl, for not knowing.

Liam has faced seasons of despondency and anxiety. These too have been a predatory and stalking enemy. I have not completely understood his need for quietness and sometimes days of solitude. I have wanted to help him get on his feet through sheer determination, upbeat encouragement, and motivation. I have placed my trust in medication. Try it. Take it. Believe in it. Why would it not work? I have not let him be because I did not know. He needs alone time, more so than the "average" (what is average anymore?) young man and I have not understood until now. I apologize, kind and winsome son of mine.

Recently we had a gathering in our home. I was not feeling well enough but the situation presented itself, so we proceeded. Six adults and two preschoolers in our home for almost two hours is nothing, or so it once was. At the halfway mark, I walked over to Liam and looked him in the eye and said, "I get you now. I understand your need for silence. Noise can be crushing and inescapable and I'm about to lose my mind right now."

He said, "Really mom? Me too. It's taking everything I have to stay right here in this room and not leave. I'm telling myself these are people I love and I need to be here, but it is so hard."

Christine has taught me life lessons as well. The outer layers of ourselves we believe must be projected to the world are often what rubs thin first, exposing the raw honesty embedded and bound beneath. It is not an option to leave loved ones when their lives are vulnerable from tenuous strands that have moved in and laid claim. Individuals may have hidden or dismissed a wound for so long they no longer acknowledge its venomous capacity for destruction. The weight of the burden may become the new normal. Attractive and eye-catching covers don't always tell the true story; and does anyone ever live happily ever after? The best books are ones where characters undergo transformation by addressing a challenge, fighting through, and making a difference in their world.

I am learning to extend my love by listening more intently. Everyone needs courage for whatever battle they may be facing. I now aspire to meet others at their point of need in a humble gesture of reaching out. I am learning to accept myself and others for who they are, not for who I wish they would be.

Random Thought:

We cannot help another without first having humility.

81
MEET ME AFTER SLIME

The front door burst open and little E and Z raced full force into the living room. Barely holding onto a big box, they squealed in delight as they ran their sentences on top of each other. I could not decipher every word but a few phrases surfaced: "It's for us, Mommy bought on vacation, can we make it, this is the best day of my life!"

"Oh wow, come and let me see," I urged.

Turning the box, I read "LET'S MAKE SLIME" and feigned an exaggerated gasp. "Shall we do this now?"

"YES, YES, YES!" they yelled in unison.

"Can you two open the box and let's see what is inside."

They pulled out the contents and set them on the table, along with the directions.

"Let me get my glasses first," I said, "so I can read the words."

A few moments later with the instructions in hand, I read the various kinds of slime that we could make. Foam slime, glitter slime, smelly slime, neon slime, squishy slime. Oh, the possibilities were thrilling. We got right down to business. Ingredients were measured precisely, stirred in a teacup, and kneaded like bread dough before it success-fully turned into the desired consistency. The delight on their faces was priceless as we procured the makings of slime. When Claire came over a littler later, the contagious sounds of laughter and fun spilled into the room once again.

"Mommy, come see what we made! We did it; WE made slime!"

The next morning, walking through that same room but alone this time, I smiled as I remembered the impromptu craft bash. The hour of slime was a joyful and charismatic highlight of our day.

"Dear God, thank you for children, their loving and joyful nature, their eagerness to please, and their delight in the world around them. Thank you for opening my eyes to see and embrace their passion in finding such thrill in life's discoveries. Thank you for their example of what true living – filled with joy and anticipation – can mean. Thank you for the blessing of slime yesterday."

82
MEET ME AT PROMOTION

I climbed into bed the night before my last day with students and thought, "I've had a joyful and active day with the end of the year activities that concluded with a fantastic Talent Show. Many inspirational students participated by sharing their passions with a captive audience. I was invigorated to walk on an unpretentious walking track, which lead to a beautiful pond afterwards. Sunshine, activity, and purpose. My day was complete."

Ouch, turn. Toss, move. Turn over. Groan. More pillows. Turn again. Different pillows. Sleep interrupted. Move again. Varying pillow placements. Now fully awake I realize my left leg and hip are in a sciatic nerve spasm which is occurring with my pulse. Oh great. I move to the floor. More experimentations in positions. In exasperation, I climb aboard a huge pillow which cradles my pelvic bones as it offers some curvature to that area, position both legs perfectly straight while holding my feet at 90 degrees with more pillows, and lower my head onto another pillow; my head is lower than my belly area. Unnatural, and not truly comfortable, but finally the nerve stilled and I drifted back to sleep.

6:15 am – the alarm. Ugghhhhh! I wasn't ready to wake up.

My last school day was today, and I have enjoyed assisting with promotional exercises and the reception which followed through the years. I stumble into the bathroom, drunken from lack of sleep. "You are NOT going to win," I tell my body. "I AM. YOU ARE NOT RUINING THIS DAY." So with a pretty dress, jewelry, hair done right and more makeup than usual under the sunken eyes, I'm off to the kitchen to grab a cup of coffee. My favorite these days is a combo of black coffee beans mixed with chicory, brewed, and laced with French Cream to soften and sweeten my morning ritual.

I arrive to school a little later than usual: 7:30 am; but after all, this is the last day. Not much to prepare. No computer labs to start up. No announcements running on the flat screens. No final worksheet or test papers to copy for the teachers. No more books to check out. Alice Cooper's musical rendition is playing in my mind.

I spend my morning in the hall greeting students and accepting the occasional found book that is finally returned. In my office at 8:30 am, I pick up the phone for the last time and press "All Call" and proceed with both flag salute pledges to the United States and to our state, and then extend an invitation for a moment of silence. I contribute a few more announcements and then with sincerity remind all students to have a safe and fun-filled summer. I've dispensed morning announcements for 19 years. This is my last time doing so.

Moving on, I go into the auditorium and visit with a former principal who has returned to present a special award. I then greet our guest speaker who was a student here eight years ago. It is thrilling to see former students stand out and succeed in the community and make our world a better place. This cycle of renewal with the next generation makes me feel proud. I had a hand in this.

The program begins with a warm salutation and followed by the request to listen to a student as she sings "The Star-Spangled Banner." I am captivated by my young friend as she steps forward from the audience, climbs the stairs in pumps and glides with perfect posture and grace to the center of the stage. She collects herself and with perfect pitch and timing, begins to sing the anthem acapella. The audience, out of respect, has risen to their feet and a hush of genuine admiration hovers as she sings on and on. She has an operatic voice with a slight reverberation as she strikes the highest notes with ease. The crowd is mesmerized. This student has attended our school nine months and this is the first time we have known of this melodic talent she possesses. How passionately she shares it with us. She is a reflective and quiet student who stands apart from others in the way she carries herself, her interest in academics and current events, her ease with speaking with adults and maturation. Her wardrobe selection conveys a high profile; her style is characteristically vintage but perfect for her.

Today she has chosen an exclusive red dress with pleated skirt, a camisole jacket and has adorned her hands with diminutive white gloves, which are both vogue and sophisticated. She is chic and fashionable and is clearly in charge of the moment. Until she isn't. As the next passage proceeds her voice falters. She struggles to reach the highest of high notes, but she knows with sadness in her heart that she will not be finishing the anthem. She stops and stands perfectly still, then turns away from the audience. We are caught in the spell of the moment and wish so desperately for her to regain confidence and command of her voice. We wait. As a few moments pass without a sound, we applaud her efforts and are inspired by her courage. She tried something none of us were willing to do. A principal on stage offers a loving embrace, and then lifts a hand as if to say, sing with us. With reverend voices in the auditorium, we finish the anthem: "and the rocket's red glare, the bombs bursting in air, gave proof through the night that our flag was still there"....until we finish.

She returns to her end seat on the second row. As I stand at the back of the auditorium, I watch and wait to see if anyone goes to provide a comforting word. The program continues onward with award presentations but my eyes are on her white gloves as they gently wipe away tears. I am holding a paper napkin from the reception table; I fold it pensively and walk to the front of the auditorium and kneel next to her. We lean in towards each other as I place it in her gloved hand, and whisper "I love you. That was beautiful and it doesn't matter. I promise, it doesn't matter."

The promotional exercises continued until completion. I hope she knows what she did took courage but, more so, it brought one thousand people together in unison as we sang deliberately and then specifically finished for her. It was a beautiful juncture. I hope she knows she made a positive impact even when she thought she had failed.

Later that evening I continue to reflect on this experience and wonder how it will inspire me in the Game of Life in my next positional point. Do I have a talent to share? Do I have the courage to step up even in the face of an unknown outcome? Will I prepare myself for the task at end by spending hours with thoughtful reflection, practice, mindset and other things needed to accomplish my goals? Will I have the grace to accept loss or what I may perceive as failure if things don't turn out as expected? Will I sense the love and community of others as they stand with me on my good days and even into the darkest nights? Will I treasure the opportunities that I am given?

Thank you, cherished friend, for showing me the way.

83
MEET ME AS I RETHINK TIME

C ompromise and customizing tasks to my body and abilities were necessary. The weight of a gallon of milk was often difficult. Carrying a pot of scalding water to empty into the kitchen sink ten steps away was not possible. "I need your help" was the standard when preparing spaghetti this year. Other changes came and without notice from others.

Lightening the load was a necessity. I exchanged a stylish leather bag for a crocheted wicker handbag. I substituted the leather carryon for a fabric one. I eliminated a few keys on my keychain. Instead of four tubes of lipstick, I selected one to go into my purse. These little subtle changes added up to a noticeable difference in weight.

My watch was a gift while on a luscious business trip to Jamaica. At the close of the convention, spouses who had attended were given a gift as a token of the company's appreciation. I had received a beautiful bangle chain type watch. For almost five years I wore this watch and appreciated the value of the generous gift.

But as my life began to swirl in a different direction with the coming of my retirement, I tucked away this watch on my dressing table. I didn't need to monitor my life by the clock so much and the watch seemed heavy on my arm now. It was also an object that no longer brought me joy but a slight sense of sorrow. "No more big trips," I thought. "Will I ever use my passport again? When will I see a real, salt in your eye, expansive from east to the west, aqua blue ocean again?" As if to prod me even further, here it was June and as I read

Facebook posts, friends were posting photos of themselves on a beach. Ugggghhhh, I couldn't get away from it!

Was the problem envy or time? Not envy – I was happy they were enjoying their summer vacations in paradise. How could time be a problem?

After brooding for a few days, I realized I wasn't sure what to do with the time looming ahead for me. I was a now a non-working, unlikely to be employed again, stay at home lady of the house. I was in unfamiliar territory and it was sobering. Having purpose and making my time count is an essential element of life but how was I to revamp it for my new season of life?

One morning I woke up and next to the coffee maker was a blue pouch from a jewelry store. I turned to my husband and asked, "Do you know how this got here?" With a priceless look on his face, Luke answered, "Yes, I got it for you. I was unclear of your last day of work, so I've been waiting to see if you were going in or not. Inside the bag is my retirement gift to you!" That perked me up. Inside was a beautiful, lightweight watch. He went on to say he thought it was just the thing I needed. Even though I had retired, I needed to keep up with things.

Luke is a time keeper and is on time wherever he goes. This watch reflected how important knowing the time of day was to him, and he was sharing that passion with me. I clasped it onto my wrist and thought, "Yes, time is still important to me, too. I may not know what each day will hold but did I ever? Wasn't I adapting my life to others, to situations and emergencies, and to life's adventures that cropped up unexpectedly? I'm still me and I still have 24 hours in which to measure my life with."

How can I measure time? Years before, Christine and I shared the love of a musical entitled *Rent*. The lyrics from "Seasons of Love" were still right on.

84
MEET ME ON A CAREER PATH

The confirmation of Hip Dysplasia was both a relief in knowing the cause of my inflexibility, but disappointing as well. My pelvic floor muscles would have an even harder time relaxing because they would continue to pull inappropriately. Maybe forever. I cannot grasp this and don't accept my affliction must be forever. Having a solution-minded attitude is the name of the game.

The PA who shared the findings on the x-ray was sensitive to my needs and patiently went through medical details with us. The only remarkable thing that happened in the office was I hugged him tight and wept quietly after the diagnosis. Confirmation is a good thing; it removes guilt that I may have caused this. But where do I go from here? With a smile he said, "Walking was good." YEA YEA YEA!!! I would have been heartbroken if he had said no. "Yes, walking one mile a day, not too fast. You don't want to strain and cause a labral tear – TRULY, you DON'T WANT THAT," he said. I'm convinced. Strolling it is.

A month later there I was in the mall, strolling and eyeing the windows. One poster caught my eye: "CAREERS that FIT" – apply online. I retracted my steps and examined it a second time. The graphic artist who designed this would be stunned by what I read into his marketing strategy: "I need to set up a CAREER that FITS me!" I continued to brainstorm. "I may need a job description. No one would be applying for this career but me. I had no competition but myself. Was I up for the challenge?"

I finished the indoor lap but continued to ponder this new concept of a career designed just for me. My work ethic started early. My first job was babysitting as a twelve-year-old girl. I was to supervise two children for about six hours: one used a bottle and ate baby food and the other was about four years old. I was given the instructions for nap time, shown how to turn the old gas stove on with matches (we used electric at our house but I showed no fear) and then offhandedly was told to make macaroni and cheese for lunch. Thankfully, my mom came a few hours later; she helped me light the stove to prepare the boiling water for the macaroni. Up until that time, the only thing I had baked was slice and bake cookies. That poor mother most definitely had needed an afternoon off or else she had tunnel vision on my babysitting abilities. Either way, the job was accomplished with happy and well-fed children who were asleep when she returned. I earned about 50 cents an hour and was proud of it.

My second job was a step up the following year. The owners of a local diner and gift shop needed someone to "pour coffee" and ring up sales. Was I available after school for a few hours? "Sure!" my parents enthusiastically exclaimed and then shared the opportunity with me. "What? Are you kidding me?" I was in the fall semester of eighth grade and this was going to greatly interfere with afterschool social time with friends. But being responsible, I went. My first day I realized this was going to be another hurdle as it was not simply pouring coffee. It was brewing the coffee, creating malts and milkshakes, preparing grilled cheese sandwiches and a few other things. My first malt ended up on the floor; how was I to know the lid must be fastened? We didn't own a blender so this was foreign to me. But I was nice and the customers no doubt took pity on me. I discovered receiving tips was fun money none of my friends had. At the end of each day, the owner opened the older cash register with buttons and levers and took out a few dollars for me. On days he left early, I earned the privilege of retrieving my own money and then locking up the store.

From there, I hoed sugar beets two weeks for a local farmer (worst job ever), more babysitting, typing and clerical, pharmacy tech, sales (retail and home pyramid type sales), afterschool care in my home, corporate daycare teacher, sixth grade science teacher, library assistant, and my last career was as a resource specialist.

The word retirement and chronic pain used in the same sentence was nothing to celebrate. I was at a tug of war in both mind and body. I usually held it together but alone in the shower the tears often flowed unashamedly. This new "Careers that Fit" plan was all about the new me but I didn't know who I was, what I was capable of, and what my long-term goals would be. My optimistic spirit had waned over the year. Hence, my first objectives: have more trust, less fear, and develop more joy. My boss was God Himself, Jesus if you will, and although I couldn't see him, I knew he would walk with me on this new career path. I believe opportunities will open and He will give me courage to step into situations I may feel unqualified or unable to do on my own. This might be the toughest career of my life.

Successful people consistently read, give compliments, embrace change, forgive others, talk about ideas, continually learn new things, accept responsibility, have a sense of gratitude, and set goals to develop new life plans. So far, so good. I could do these. This time around, there would be no specific clock in time, and no time monitoring of any kind in fact. There would be goal-setting but no formal evaluations. The product was ME and the procedural plan involved internal work. My strongest assets were listening, reading, and serving others. However, lifting heavy boxes is difficult now and I must frequently switch positions. I don't wear heels and I need to rest more. But these conditions had absolutely no effect on the successfulness of my possible new career.

I love Wikipedia's definition of a career: "A career is an individual's journey through learning, work, and other aspects of life." On-the-go training, confidence, and a plan for success were going in the toolbox for this new career title: Journey Walker. I won't always understand the path; I may need to look inward and be prepared to face dark aspects of this journey. Am I a tribe of one? I could reach out to others who are facing challenges, share our victories and train my eyes to discover new truths for life. This road may lead straight into wilderness, or level terrain, or wind itself up a steep path. I will find fulfillment as I get up and go. With faith, I trust in Him who will guide me in the right direction.

This was not my original game plan but sometimes you have to drop the what ifs, let go, free fall, and have faith that your life isn't about to shatter upon impact. My new career path will be my opened parachute. I will learn to step out and hold on.

Isaiah 41:10

Do not fear, for I am with you; do not be afraid, for I am your God. I will strengthen you; I will help you; I will hold onto you with My righteous right hand. (Christian Standard Bible)

85
MEET ME IN THANKFULNESS

I am thankful for a vocation that allowed me to get up out of the chair, be alone, be with people, bend, move, talk, be quiet, be of service to others, and was enjoyable at the same time. All this every single day. I survived this final year of my career because it was a perfect fit.

I am thankful for my husband who in his 20s believed we ought to begin saving for retirement. We invested 10% of our income and his employer matched it. Without this reserved investment, I would not be able to retire earlier than at the standard age of 62.

I am thankful for sweet hearted and laughing grandchildren who live close by.

I am thankful for my three children and one son-in-love who are unique, talented, motivated, creative and make our lives complete.

I am thankful my father is alive and healthy. My mother has gone on and I have her memories, but having a father 70 miles away is a bonus in life.

I am thankful for my two brothers, a sister by marriage, and the varied aspects of life and joy they provide to my heart.

I am thankful for warm days and spring flowers.

I am thankful we have a boat and I can comfortably ride in it, and the lake is only 18 minutes away.

I am thankful for my ladies' class with caring members who have brought dear friendship into my life.

I am thankful for the treasure of my three college friends, the Bon Temps sisterhood. Without them I would be lost.

I am thankful for my Devotional Guide and Bible that anchors my life in times of fear and uncertainty.

I am thankful I still look healthy and stylish.

I am thankful I have a creative spirit.

I am thankful my husband and I have a shared vision of helping others, especially the underdog and those needing our charity.

I am thankful God has a plan for my life.

I am thankful for good memories.

I am thankful Luke remains loyal through this season of uncertainty.

I am thankful for a caring team of health professionals whom I trust.

I am thankful I have the assurance of Heaven.

86
MEET ME ON MY ANNIVERSARY

Today marks the one-year anniversary of my relationship with pelvic floor therapy. One year ago today I lay in the backseat of my husband's F-150 pickup truck. Numerous pillows softened the vibrations of the vehicle. Our drive was 90 miles each way and I have never looked forward to an appointment the way I did this one. I had waited six weeks and counted down the days. Initially I had been told it would be an easy process to be referred to this clinic. However, due to factors that slowed the process, those 50 plus days of waiting were emotionally draining. When a person is in pain, each day is a long test of endurance.

I am nervous. I relive the past. I feel off and I have for days in anticipation of this anniversary. I cannot overlook this day but I'm at a loss as to know what to do. How does one celebrate or honor a day like today? I can either dwell on the past or think of the present. I chose joy for today instead of being a "Debbie Downer." Luke and I made plans to honor the day with something we love, and that meant a trip to the lake. That afternoon in a swimsuit, wearing sunglasses, and with a thick application of sunscreen I stretched out and atop the comfy cushions of the boat. The warm sun was welcomed. I listened to the gulls as they flew overhead. The lapping water from the gentle waves against the hull were destressing to me. A cool drink kept me hydrated. I was thankful to have this lake nearby, our own boat, and a husband who was boss when boating. He was in charge and I was grateful to turn the afternoon over to him and not fret about one thing. I let time pass.

I recently adopted a conscious mindset. During moments of anxiety or when I am sad, disappointed, or fearful, I concentrate on letting time pass. This mantra removes the pressure to solve the problem immediately. It also diffuses frantic feelings that bubble up from the inside when I have lost control. I am not successful in every situation to let time pass, but like anything worth doing, I agreed with myself to work at it until it became a part of my routine.

Random Thought:

Thank you, Father, for allowing me to simplify my day.

87
MEET ME ON A GOOD DAY

My face smiles. I help others today.

My mind opens to new opportunities.

I do not dwell on pain. I can sit.

I may be able to kneel, squat, stroll, or bend without too much discomfort.

I don't use the heating pad today.

I only take one hot shower.

I eat three times today.

I am pleasant.

I can read a chapter in a book without losing interest.

I feel happy and am cautiously optimistic.

A few more chores get accomplished.

I am not chilled to the bone.

I am hopeful. I LOVE good days.

88
MEET ME AND THE BLOOD TEST

I hate waiting. Seriously, how long does it take to order a blood test? Honestly, she doesn't know how long I have been waiting.

I have been asking and waiting for months. Initially I asked for a blood test to determine my hormone levels and was told it was more accurate to listen to symptoms instead. "Hormones fluctuate," they said, "and unless you do multiple blood tests, a true determination is impossible." My symptoms grew worse and still no one tested my blood. Blood is the key. Why doesn't anyone want to look deeply into my blood to discover the missing code? Something may be there.

Doctor G agrees to test my blood after I ask the receptionist on the phone. What am I looking for? Primarily, IF this dysfunction was the result of a hormonal imbalance, I want to know where I stand on hormones now. Do I need to increase or taper off? Will my body begin to produce them if an imbalance is found or do I need supplements the rest of my life? What kind – chemical or biological?

I also question if I have a vitamin B12 deficiency. A study shows women with pelvic pain dysfunction have deficiencies in vitamins B1, B6, B12, and D. Specifically, a deficiency in vitamin B12 causes nerve damage due to lack of oxygen. This is presented in pins and needles, electric shocks throughout the body, short-term memory loss, and vision problems (all of which I have).

Please call me to confirm my bloody BLOOD TEST! I'm dying to know.

L

A

T

E

R

Sigh, I got the test results and my levels were normal.

Background: www.ncbi.nlm.nih.gov/pcm/articles/PMC33492521/

Nutritional deficiencies and metabolic disorders are not uncommon among women with MFPP but may be overlooked by medical practitioners as an underlying contributor to CPP. Deficiencies of vitamins B1, B6, and B12, folic acid, vitamin C and D, iron, magnesium and zinc have all been associated with chronic MTrPs (Dommerholt, Bron & Franssen 2006). In people with chronic MTrPs, 16% have insufficient B12 levels, while 90% lack proper vitamin D. Months of treatment may be required before levels become normal (Dommerholt et al.).

MFPP (Myofascial Pelvic Pain); CPP (Chronic Pelvic Pain); MTrPs (Myofascial trigger Points)

Random Thought:

What is my next step?

89
MEET ME AND JACK

O nce upon a time, a friend who was incredibly spunky got sick with a cold. She drove to the minor emergency clinic and just as the doctor instructed her to say "ahhh," her face began to look different. Apparently, she was having a stroke! Rushing to the hospital for a stroke which then turned into a brain tumor, which needed operating, was too much! My fast-acting friend called in her troops and declared, we need to get rid of Earl, the tumor. With her head held high, she threatened Earl within an inch of his life to get out as words from the Dixie Chicks bellowed with "Good Bye Earl." Having a sense of humor was contagious and we sent our sentiments for Earl to back off, leave her alone, and get the heck out of there, Earl!

Ray Charles is iconic and I have decided to adopt one of his best musical renditions as my theme song. "Hit the Road, Jack" plays in my head with a twist of fun and irony as I speak directly to my dysfunction whom I have affectionately named "Jack."

"Jack, I'm sick of you!"

Jack has lived with me for a year and half and it's time we part ways. And to drive the idea home even further, four times Ray rings out to not come back. No more.

"Hey Jack, are you LISTENING to me?"

90

MEET ME AND MY INTUITIVE FRIEND

O ur ladies class had been studying thankfulness. Our facilitator asked, "Has there ever been a time in which you were overwhelmingly thankful for a situation?"

"Well, yes," my heart thundered in my chest. I spoke up. I had no alternative. "This has been the worst year of my life. As you know I have had a muscular issue. You can see I sit in a chair which is different from yours. But a few months ago, I began to feel a bit better so I then tapered off some of my medication. Through the weeks, I have become cautiously optimistic that I'm improving. But now I'd like to sweep that aside and say I know God is healing me."

Stunned silence. Then my intuitive friend looked intently into my eyes and asked, "How did you express thanks as you were going through this past year or does one need to wait for restoration to be thankful?" I stumbled around and said, "This past year brought me to the foundation of my life, to have new eyes to see the basics and realize God was with me. He showed Himself to me through others, through my family; He helped me make it through this past year."

Then I said, "You might have given me this question earlier so I could think about it first!"

Hours later, I am still pondering this question, and I have now come up with a more articulate answer:

"This has been the worst 17 months of my life. I was drowning. There was no ending to the pain and physical suffering I encountered on a minute-by-minute basis many days. I begged God for answers, for strength, for a way out. The pain was intense and dominated all senses. I was miserable and for many days and weeks, I lived one moment to the next. The first year of this affliction was spent in research, coping, sleeping to block out pain, and trying to carry on with the basics of my life. The agony showed in my face, gait, and posture. My eyes lost their sparkle. I struggled. I aged into an old senior adult, or so it seemed.

God held my hand and listened to my cries, not in the way I wanted a timely answer to be, but He shed His presence in my dark life by presenting Himself in small miracles. He gave me peace. He lessened the pain. He allowed me the dignity of finishing strong the course, which was set before me in my career path. I perceived his loving kindness as he brought my medical team together to care for me. He spoke to me through literature, through scripture, through friends, and nature. He put a lightness in my heart as I listened and bathed in the healing water of praise songs. He gave my mind rest. He gave me purpose by providing tasks to do – a spoken word or meaningful hug to another. He enlightened and enlarged my path and although it was a dark journey, He walked with me. I am thankful as each bend in the road shed light as to where He had been, and that His support gave me guidance. He did not design this pain for me but was there through it all. I am thankful He saw me through the worst and has promised to stay with me forever, with many good things to come."

In answer to your question, sweet friend:

"I'm ashamed to say that I do not know how to express thanks in times of suffering, but I am learning."

91

MEET ME WITH LOSSES AND GAINS

Items and services purchased for the pelvic pain journey:

FROM December 2015 – August 2017

2 Heating pads and a car adaptor	65
Leggings	100
Long Dresses/skirts from Goodwill	150
Walgreens medications	1200
Compounded medications	225
Mail order Valium compound	432
Massage tools	175
Acupuncture	2335
Massage – 26 sessions	1270
Chiropractic visits	235
Underwear	175
Sitz bath and Epsom salts	28

Indoor hammock	125
Rubber water trough	60
Various creams	55
TENS machine and pads	104
Specialist visits and 24 PT sessions	2343
Dr. B, C, D, E, & G copays	200
X-Ray	14
4 Books and relaxation CDS	85
Oxalate supplements at health food store	91
Seat cushions and a toilet seat	100
Hotel with Jacuzzi bath	238
Gas for PT	475
Tolls for PT	425
Go Commandos cotton patches	52
Laptop	430
Smooth Tea for constipations – 5 boxes	25
Tests and surgery in Dec of 2015	1052
SUBTOTAL	11,887

Suburban with Magnetic Ride Control	
and nitrogen filled tires	$40,000
Taxes and Registration	750
TOTAL	$52,637
MENTAL STRESS	Incalculable
EMOTIONAL STRESS	Incalculable
PAIN AND SUFFERING	Incalculable

What have I GAINED?

Less micromanaging

A deeper relationship with my husband

Empathy for others

Less judgment of others

Sensitivity to suffering; motivated to help others

A deeper spiritual awakening and dependency on God

More thankfulness for things I took for granted

92

MEET ME ALONG THE SHORE

FOOTPRINTS IN THE SAND

One night I dreamed I was walking along the beach with the Lord. Scenes from my life flashed across the sky. In each, I noticed footprints in the sand. Sometimes there were two sets of footprints; other times there was only one.

During the lowest times of my life I could see only one set of footprints, so I said, "Lord, you promised me, that you would walk with me always. Why, when I have needed you most, would you leave me?"

The Lord replied, "My precious child, I love you and would never leave you. The times when you have seen only one set of footprints, it was then that I carried you."

Author Unknown

93
MEET ME DEEP IN CONVERSATION

O livia: "Are you stretching out like you were doing? Your inner right thigh was tight today."

Me: "Yesterday and today before I came in, I walked two miles. Do you think that has something to do with it?"

Olivia: "Two miles total or two miles each day?"

Me: "Two each day."

Olivia: "No, that's appreciable you are walking that far. We don't want you to move backward in achievement. But were you stretching afterwards?"

Me: "No, I didn't do that after each time but I'll start."

Olivia (moving towards the padded flooring area): "Here, like this. Stretch out those inner thighs and hips. Remember to also relax during the day and let your legs gently open, without straining."

Me: "Yes, I will start doing that again."

Olivia: "You are coming back in two weeks, right?"

Me: "Yes, and I want to hear all about your trip next time. Going to Nashville during the eclipse is going to be amazing. Did I tell you I'm taking a trip, too?"

Olivia: "Where are you going?"

Me: "Destin, Florida. In four days. I'm going by myself."

Olivia: "Wow, that's something. By yourself? Why Destin?"

Me: "Luke and I planned for about a year to go as a celebration of my retirement and the ending to all this. The trip didn't seem possible a few months ago so we dropped it. But I asked him two weeks ago if he would mind if I went. I'm feeling stronger and I need to go. You know this has been such an unexpected year."

Olivia: "Yes, it has. And he is okay with you going alone?"

Me: "Well, he said, 'what if I say no?' And I said I would be disappointed and sad. He murmured that he didn't want that, so go ahead and make the airline reservations."

Olivia: "Well, what are you going to do?"

Me: "I'm going to enjoy the beach and relax. I'm going to write and read. Ummm." Pause. "Olivia, I have something to tell you."

Olivia (looking directly into my face, bewildered): "What is it?"

Me: "Do you remember I planned on writing a book about pelvic pain? I'm going to Destin to write the book."

Olivia (with smiles): "That's great! Your own journey. I have not seen another memoir of someone with pelvic floor dysfunction on the market. When you said you were going to read and write in Destin, were you talking about writing this book?"

Me (shaking my head yes): "I'm almost finished with it.

Olivia (shocked): "Oh my gosh. Can I tell Dr. Hannah?"

Me: "Yes. Of course! I'm going to change your names and the identity of this clinic. I would need corporate permission and it might be drawn out, and then they would most likely say no in the end. So, I'm going to change identifiers to protect myself."

Olivia: "That's a good idea. You can call me Olivia."

I turned to go and she asked softly, "How will you end the book?"

Me: "I haven't figured that out yet."

May the words of my mouth and the thoughts of my heart be pleasing to You. Psalm 19:14

(The Living Bible)

94
MEET ME IN THE END

If I take hormones the rest of my life

If I only use water to bathe

If I stay away from the gossiping crowd

If I chose to walk away.

If I stretch out my legs and my hips every day

Will my muscles succumb to their bands?

Will my bones remember the way they were made

When my body obeys its commands?

If I keep improving my mind and my flesh

Will they eventually learn to relax?

How much longer will this role that I play

Be a part of my attainable tasks?

If I take the right dosage of medicine and herbs

If I find I'm deficient in some

Will my tissues regain the extension they had?

Will my moments in Hell fade away?

If I walk with a gait that is healthy and whole

If I sleep on a warm heating pad

Will my pain dissipate and the tears I've withheld

Make a difference in life up ahead?

I hope and I pray that this thing goes away

And I want to live life with a smile

Engaged in life; finding the good in each day

And without an offense in my world.

But I know it is truly impossible

We all have our burdens we bear

The key is to open our hearts in true love

and to willingly care and to share.

If granted one wish for today it would be

That I might possibly have

A life I courageously sought 'til the end

To be strong, and whole, and to win.

The prerequisite is to focus on you

and to offer my soul from the start

As you travel your road may I, too come along

More able we'll be than apart.

95

MEET ME IN DESTIN, FINALLY

S unday Morning. I am sitting on white sands with the endless ocean before me. My hands cup the grains as they flow effortlessly through my fingers and drain again and again upon the unblemished beach. I close my eyes and whisper the words: "This is real." I cannot believe I am here. Nor can I believe I have battled pelvic pain for 18 months. Both are surreal. I have a hard time processing the "now." I am more of the not now but later type of girl. However, I savor this moment; I do not want to miss one stroke of awareness. I am cognizant of my appointment to be at the sea.

Groups of two and three, and families of more are gathered here today. As I swivel in a 360 degree from my point of reference on the beach I observe an abundance of joy. A young baby floats with a thoughtfully placed umbrella shade over his cradle in the surf as his momma holds tight to this pint-sized tubal watercraft. A circle of girlfriends chattered and listened attentively to one another. No cell phones in sight. A couple in love hold hands. They are senior adults; with the loving touch of their hands and many years as evidenced in their care for one another, they venture out into the waves. Together they go and laughingly the woman falls into the surf as its power knocks her off her center. The sweet provision of love is rendered within the gentle embrace as he lifts her to her feet and they go onward to see what awaits.

Bikinis, fishnet cover-ups, and long tunics to guard the sun are in vogue. All aspects of apparel are welcome here. I see a plethora of color from the umbrellas placed strategically in the sand to the beach towels and distinctive sun bonnets. Playing along the seashore, swimming in the waters, reading in the shade and even the occasional napping individual are a few of the scattering of people who display their agendas. We have all come here to enjoy and our expectations for R & R (rest and relaxation) are high.

Walking out into the emerald green water, my eyes catch the flittering movement of sea perch as they swim and play together. Elongated transparent fish also dip just below the surface. An occasional one of substantial size glides by and I gasp in surprise.

As I tilt my head upward, I gaze at a colorful object in the air and then smile at the recollection of my first parasailing jaunt along the beaches of Ixtapa, Mexico thirty years ago. "Could I go out again?" or "am I content to watch others fly high and allow me this present time around to observe the casual beauty of their sails?" A few solitary individuals have rented surfboards, boogie boards and kayaks in hopes of venturing out further with the eternal quest of discovering "what is out there." Fishing boats on the horizon are stalled with heavy anchors while white capped waves curl under the bow. I suppose one may catch my scrumptious supper later this week at a local restaurant.

The warm sunshine and healing salt in the air, the roar of the surf as it crashes then washes upon the sand, and the pleasant sounds of country and western melodies which play nearby all remind me of the myriads of life's experiences as each blend seamlessly together. Our senses are aroused and we eagerly look forward to capturing a new discovery, a new insight. The gifts of the sea are revitalizing.

The wind-swept sand consists only of white grains and a few drying stalks of seaweed surfaced from the night before. No shells today. I am a bit saddened to realize if I want to leave this paradise with a beautiful seashell, I may need to buy one in a local shop across the street from my home away from home. With insight, I realize the scene in front of me with its breathtaking sea creatures, sand and surf, and glorious skies of all hues of blue and artistically sculpted clouds is more than simply a destination spot. This spectacular setting is more than shape, color, and form. The sea provides a rest for our souls in which we can lay down our burdens and just be. We have come from many places to experience keen awareness from the sea. Together, we are united. We desire to take this heightened sense of respectful beauty of the land and water back to our often mundane lifestyles of responsibilities and agendas

I see a flash of darkness out of the corner of my eye. I stand amazed. A dozen feet from where I am positioned waist high in the crystal waters I observe sea eels swimming from left to right in the waves. Snakes abhor me; yet I am transfixed as these eels make their way together down the coastline. I have no fear.

As I sit upon the sand which cradles my painful tailbone, I gently open my right hip to allow optimal stretching. Others are lying, bending, crouching, splashing, standing, swimming and gliding, resting, dancing, strolling, and skipping. The gulls call out from overhead as they cascade from up above to below in hopes of fetching a crumb. I see no right or wrong way to be here. The sea diminishes all self-subscribed protocols. I want to relish life.

I detect a nibble on my left leg and smile as I search for the fish that courageously crept up on me. Alas, no fish are nearby but instead those nerve endings are firing. This is my new normal, yet with renewed understanding, I focus my attention on the sea instead of on me. This is what I will take back instead of a handsome shell. I will honor the sea by observing its beauty and accept the intricacies that make me the one of a kind person I am. I will not live as if I am entangled anymore but view my anatomy as an elaborate workmanship which even defies medical knowledge. I am perfect the way I am. I recommit myself to love. I desire to open my mind to opportunities and blessings around me. Stepping away from a challenge will not be an option. I release fear. I ask for a grateful heart to reflect grace and refreshment to others. Allow me to share the journey of growth.

I pledge to seek evidences I am woven into the pattern of Your creation. I am not in Destin alone; all Life is with me. My souvenir from this pilgrimage is this revelation. Destin has disclosed my Destiny. I will relish the sea in me.

August 19-24, 2017

With Love

Amy

96
MEET ME AND A GOAL

September 5, 2017

Olivia: "You have now met your original goals. It's time to set new ones. What would you like to work towards doing next?"

97
MEET ME AND MY OPTIONS

R eaders may voice concern as to why I didn't do this or that, or ask for a certain medication or obtain a second opinion.

1. The nearest physical therapist and gynecologist who specialize in pelvic floor therapy are 90 miles away.

2. Claire, a Registered Nurse, shared with colleagues about my dysfunction (with permission); no one had heard of this.

3. My new family practice physician, Dr. G, was glad to receive a phone call from Dr. Hannah to clarify the complications and treatment options for treating pelvic floor dysfunction. I wanted my team to work together, and communication is the key. If a medical doctor is not aware of the availabilities for treatment, what does this say about the public in general? It's the worst secret out there.

4. Possibly no one mentioned the option you are thinking of.

5. Maybe I didn't discover a technique, tool, or this, that, or the other during my own research.

6. You may have benefitted from time. Maybe the option you are using now had not been field tested during my duration of hell.

7. The use of Botox or nerve blocks may be options in the future should I need them, but at this point they are unnecessary.

8. Distance and time. It was not considered a pleasure trip to drive to any more appointments than necessary.

9. Although money wasn't a key role in choosing health care options, my expenses did require budgeting.

I can only imagine what my coworkers might say, considering they would read a book of this nature. I guess out of curiosity they might!

"Why didn't you tell me?"

"You looked fine!"

This is how I did it, my dear friends.

1. I wore makeup, fixed my hair, and wore stylish clothes to avoid looking sick.

2. My students did most of the manual work.

3. I rarely sat.

4. I worked on many individual projects.

5. I carried one object at a time.

6. I often stood outside for a few minutes to meditate.

7. I much preferred to listen to you talk rather than discuss my life.

98
MEET ME IN THE PHOTO ALBUM

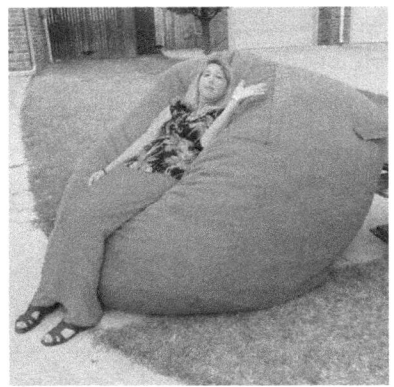

The enormous beanbag

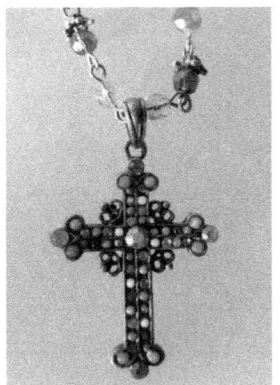

The spontaneous gift

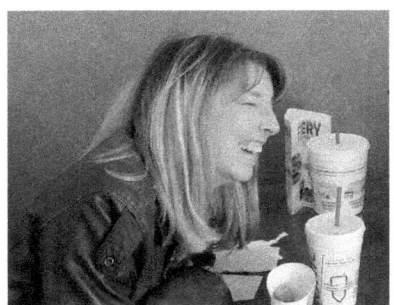

Laughter is the best medicine

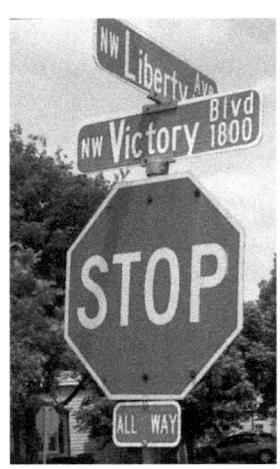

Standing on the
corner of Victory

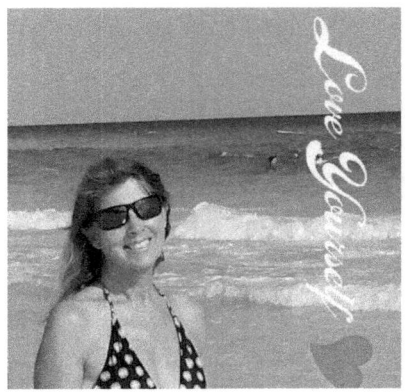

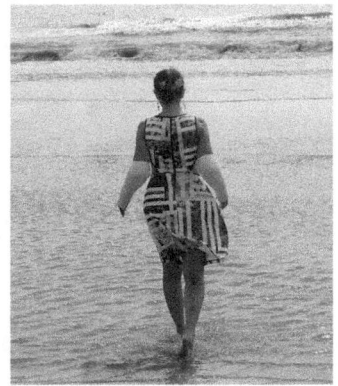

On the beach at Destin, Florida

Moving forward despite
fractured elbows

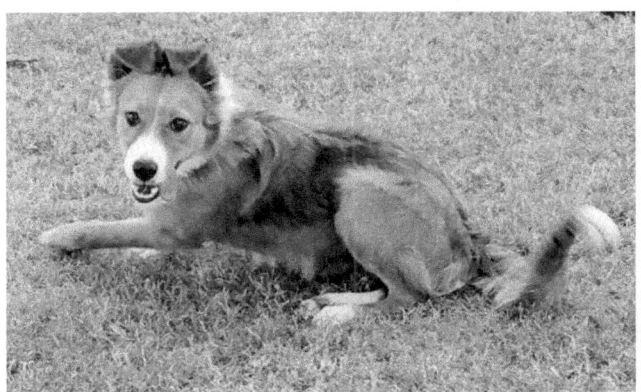

"Journey" – the new dog that adopted me

99
MEET ME INCOGNITO

As I sift through blogs this year, I am amazed how many authors share freely with gut-wrenching stories of their experiences with pain and life, but write incognito. Maybe they don't want to be permanently attached to their thoughts on paper, or in cyberspace. Often, people simply refer to themselves with first names. The norm online when dealing with chronic and discreet situations that belong to you permit these relatively false identities.

I, too, am struggling about printing my full name on a manuscript. Is it wise to open my life to the nitty gritty, and quite embarrassing, situations I have found myself in? Will I face any negative fallout in my community? Will anyone who knows me read this months or years later be saddened or even traumatized from my story? Would it be better to name myself something different and save us all the trouble? Would it matter in the end?

New identification ideas:

#behindmysmile

#noquestionsplease

Don't say I look tired

#willthiseverend

At least you can wear jeans

#bibleversesaresavingme

I don't like belly-aching

#amyinprint

The journey goes through it

#improudofmyself

My distance goals increased as I began to "step out" more and for longer segments of time. "The Spatula Sisters" had evolved into the "Stepping Out Society" and I felt invigorated. One morning I experimented with walking uphill a short distance. So far so good. Quickening my pace and moving with gravity, I began to descend the slope. Out of nowhere, both feet caught together as in a straight-jacket, I was airborne, and then tumbled HARD onto the asphalt street. WHAT? Looking down, both shoes were tangled in a cord that had slipped on without notice. After the initial shock, and a visit to the medical clinic, I realized I had a health condition I could discuss in public now without reservation: two broken elbows! Seriously, who achieves the maneuvers necessary to produce two broken funny bones?

After eighteen months of pelvic pain, believe me, this was a breeze! Those fractured elbows would heal in the grand scheme of time, and they didn't slow this girl down. I had things to do and people to see!

100
MEET ME WITH A DISCLAIMER

- Any medical information included is based on my personal experience. For questions and concerns regarding your health or diagnosis, please consult a doctor or medical professional.

- Pelvic pain affects both men and women. This memoir is described from my point of view.

- *Meet Me: A Journey Through Pelvic Pain* is a work of nonfiction. This memoir was not embellished but is, was, and will be forever true.

- All names of persons and most institutions, as well as identifying markers have been changed to protect the good, the bad, and the ugly. Except mine.

- Personal names included were chosen with affection.

  Luke: Patron Saint of Artists; writer and physician who profiled many acts of healing in the Bible. (Husband)

  Claire: Clear. Clara Barton, pioneer who founded the American Red Cross (Daughter)

  Christine: Follower of Christ (Daughter)

  Liam: Protector (Son)

  Eduardo: Prosperous Guardian (Son-in-Law)

Cecelia: In memory of her mother and known as Patron Saint of Music (Bon Temps Friend)

Lila: In memory of her mother meaning Dark Haired Beauty (Bon Temps Friend)

Sarah: Self-chosen by the individual, meaning Noblewoman and a Lady (Bon Temps Friend)

Angela: Messenger (Technology Friend)

Bella Ruth: Beautiful Friend (Friend)

Elena: Shining Light (Friend)

Evie: Life (Chinese health and wellness friend)

Gala: One who is brave, happy and filled with peace. (Friend)

Liora: God's Gift of Light to Me (Friend)

Valerie: Strong and capable (Friend)

Melody: Song. Massage Therapy and Acupuncturist

Olivia: Self-chosen by the individual and in Latin derives from "Olive" meaning the symbol of Peace. Physical Therapy Assistant at the Pelvic Pain Clinic

Dr. Hannah: Favor and Grace. Doctor of Physical Therapy at the Pelvic Pain Clinic

Dr. A: Personal gynecologist for thirty years

Dr. B: OBGYN Doctor who performed the PAP and discovered the need for further tests

Dr. C: OBGYN Doctor within the clinic

Dr. D: OBGYN Doctor who performed all biopsies

Dr. E: OBGYN Specialist at Pelvic Pain Clinic

Dr. F: Family physician for many years

Dr. G: New local family physician

REFERENCES

Feinberg, Margaret. *Fight Back with Joy: celebrate more, regret less, stare down your greatest fears.* Worthy Publishing, 2015.

Herrera, Isa. *Ending Female Pain: A Woman's Manual: the ultimate self-help guide for women suffering from chronic pelvic and sexual pain.* Duplex Publishing, 2014.

Lauw, Adriaan, et al. Why Pelvic Pain Hurts: *Neuroscience education for patients with pelvic pain.* International Spine and Pain Institute, 2014.

Prendergast, Stephanie A., and Elizabeth H. Rummer. *Pelvic Pain Explained: what everyone needs to know.* Rowman & Littlefield, 2016.

Stein, Amy. *Heal Pelvic Pain: a proven stretching, strengthening, and nutrition program for relieving pain, incontinence, IBS, and other symptoms without surgery.* McGraw-Hill, 2009

Young, Sarah. *Jesus Calling: enjoying peace in His presence: devotions for every day of the year.* Thomas Nelson, 2011.

Why it Hurts Down There: what you need to know about Pelvic Floor Dysfunction. April 1, 2014 by Sari Harrar, Prevention, www.prevention.com/sex/understanding-pelvic-floor-dysfunction

RESOURCES

American Physical Therapy Association/Women's Health Section: https://www.apta.org

Facebook Groups related to all types of chronic pain.

Interstitial Cystitis Network: http://www.ic-network.co/forum/forum.php

InstituteForWomeninPain.com

International Pelvic Pain Society: https://pelvicpain.org

MethodistSexualWellness.com

National Vulvodynia Association: nva.org

Pelvic Health and Rehabilitation: https://www.pelvicpainrehab.com

Pelvic Pain Solutions: https://www.pelvicpainsolutions.com

Pelvic Pain Support Network: https://healthunlocked.com/pelvicpain

PracticalPainManagement.com

Women's Health Foundation: http://womenshealthfoundation.org

* Amy Watkins can be reached at turtle.tears4u@gmail.com.

I would love to hear your ideas for living a life of joy and purpose while meeting a health challenge. For those who need a friend alongside their journey, feel free to reach out to me.

Gratitude is given to Kathy Suttles
of SuttleimpressionsS Photography

CPSIA information can be obtained
at www.ICGtesting.com
Printed in the USA
BVHW05s2031300418
514824BV00019B/477/P